Back Pain

2 Manuscripts - Back Pain, Sciatica

Roger C. White

If you find this book helpful, please leave a review on Amazon here. It will help others also find this book.

AF482549

Table of Contents

Book 1 - Back Pain

Alleviate Back Pain and Start Healing Today (Simple Exercises, Remedies, and Therapy for Immediate Relief)

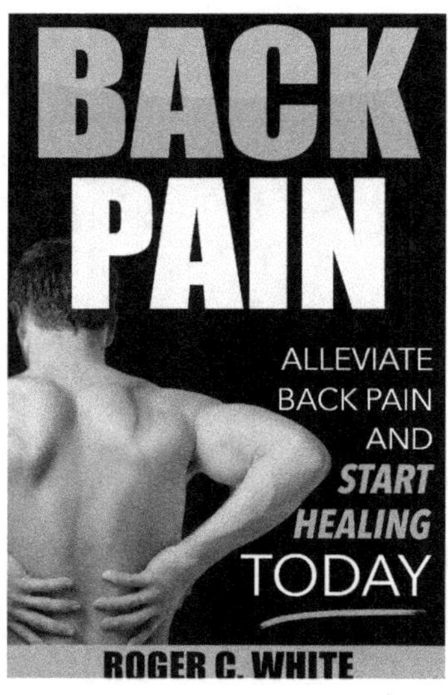

1 - Getting Started

I want to thank you and congratulate you for purchasing the book, "Back Pain".

Back Pain- A Problem that is Far Too Common

If you are afflicted by back pain, you are certainly not the only one. The majority of adults go through this specific type of pain at least once in their life. Back pain is the most common reason for disability as related to work and one of the main contributing factors to people missing work. A widespread recent survey proved that over a fourth of the adults questioned had experienced back pain in the last few months.

This is a problem that affects men and women equally, and can range from a constant, dull aching sensation to an intense and sudden pain that incapacitates the sufferer. Back pain can start suddenly as a direct result of strain, an accident, heavy lifting, or it can gradually develop from changes in the spine resulting from aging. Inactive lifestyles, which are all too common nowadays, can also pave the way for intense back pain, particularly when someone goes from getting to exercise whatsoever into a lot of exercise in a day.

There is Hope for this Affliction, no Matter Who you are

This is a widespread issue which can have many causes and vary a lot, but one common factor in all sufferers is that they want to find a way to ease this issue. In this book, we will cover some of the most common causes for back pain (to help you avoid it), along with simply exercises, stretches, and changes in lifestyle you can adopt to help this problem.

Thanks again for buying this book, I hope you enjoy it!

2 - Types and Causes of Back Pain

In order to better understand back pain, you should first understand that there are different categories for the type of pain it is possible to experience. These vary in intensity, length of time, and lasting effects. Here are the most common categories, starting with the most common of all:

- Actue Back Pain

- Sub-Scute Back Pain

- Chronic Back Pain

It is important to take a little time to explore each of these.

3 - Acute Back Pain

Shorter Lasting

The majority of back pain experienced by people is acute, meaning that it only lasts for a few days or weeks, or just in the short term. Their body is able to recover relatively quickly from acute pain.

Rarely Permanent

This type of pain has a tendency to be resolved without much hassle and doesn't leave behind any loss of abilities or permanent problems. Unlike other types of pain, they don't notice any lingering symptoms from the pain.

Disruption in Components

Most of this type of pain is of the mechanical variety, which means that something has been disrupted in the fitting together and movement of the back's components (such as the nerves, discs, muscle, or spinal cord). Rather than being the result of a deeper or underlying issue, this is more comparable to a temporary disruption in the machinery of the body.

4 - Sub-acute Back Pain

Lasts a Medium Length of Time

This pain category is a bit shorter lasting than the acute category. Typically, sufferers experience sub-acute pain for a month to a year. During this time, the pain may subside for periods or stay at a certain level continuously. Sufferers may notice that certain times of day, they pain is worse (while lying in bed, or sitting too long, for example).

Typically Heals Completely

This type of pain will most commonly resolve itself and go away, but sufferers may notice faint twinges from time to time, even months after they have healed completely. There also may be certain activities that "activate" the pain again, like intense physical activity or lifting something heavy.

5 - Chronic Back Pain

Long Lasting

Unlike the two previous categories, chronic back pain is more serious because it lasts for a year or longer. Many times, it occurs after the cause of acute pain or the initial injury has been attended to or treated by a doctor. At times, the pain may subside completely, only to show up again soon after.

It can Result from Acute Pain

About one-fifth of people who suffer acute pain in their lower back will proceed to get chronic pain after 12 months with symptoms that are persistent.

Treatment doesn't always Work: In many cases, treatment for this pain will get rid of it altogether, but for others, this pain will persist in spite of surgical or medical treatments from professionals.

6 - Back Pain, a Worsening Issue

The intensity of numbers of people who suffer from back pain has gotten worse over the years, especially since the '90s. About 20 years ago, studies showed that back pain was the sixth most burdensome health condition in the United States, but in a study conducted more recently, it had moved up to third place. This proves that the condition is getting worse and worse with time. This could be due to a variety of factors.

Increasingly Sedentary Lifestyles

One reason that back pain seems to be getting worse in American citizens is that we have increasingly inactive lifestyles. It is more and more common that people drive everywhere instead of walking, or sit at desks for long periods of time without shifting position.

In order for our muscles to get what they need to stay functioning at optimal capacity, we have to get our blood flowing regularly. Without doing this, our bodies weaken more and more with time.

Poor Nutrition

Nutrition plays a direct role in how well our bodies function. The integrity of the components of our back has a lot to do not only with how young and resilient our bodies are, but the nutrients we feed them.

The diet of the typical American is not healthy at all and is sadly devoid of the nutrients our bodies need for healthy backs and lives, in general. Nutrition is a factor that everyone suffering pain should take into consideration for healing themselves and preventing future injuries or problems.

Working Long Hours

Jobs that involve long hours, whether it be career choices that involve heavy physical labor and a lot of motion, or jobs that require you to sit eight hours a day, can contribute to the increasing back pain issue in America.

Stopping to consider whether your job is contributing to your pain is important, so you can work on making the changes you need. This could involve taking breaks more often, making sure you sit down and rest or stand up and walk when needed, and more.

The considerations listed above are just a few examples of what could be causing back pain. But in order to get to the bottom of this and make the situation better, it's important to find out more about the subject. Since lower back pain is the most common, that is what we'll focus on with this chapter.

What Components does the Lower Back Consist of?

The Lumbar Region of the Back

The lower part of the back is the most common area for pain, and is made up of the lumbar region. This consists of five different vertebrae and does most of the work for supporting the upper body's weight.

Intervertebral Discs

In between the vertebra, there are rubbery, round pads that are meant to act as absorbers of shock. These are called intervertebral discs and exist throughout the column of the spine, cushioning your bones as your upper body moves.

Ligaments and Tendons

The vertebra is held in place by ligaments which are made up of tissue bands, while the muscles are held to the spine with tendons.

Nerves

At the root of the spinal cord, there are about thirty nerve pairs, intended to control the movements of the body and act as transmitters for messages between the brain and the body.

What are some of the Main Causes of Back Pain?

Most of the pain in the back has to do with a disruption in the components listed above. In other words, the relationship between the parts is not functioning correctly. However, in a lot of other instances, pain in the lower back has to do with spondylosis. This means the typical wear and tear that happens to the spine as people age, and affects the bones, discs, and joints.

Intervertebral Degeneration of Disks in the Back

This is one of the most common factors in lower pain of the back and happens when these discs (which are usually rubbery) start to lose this quality as you age.

When someone's back is normal and healthy, these discs allow for bending, providing height, torsion, and flexion of the lower part of the back. As you grow older, these discs begin deteriorating and their ability to cushion no longer functions correctly.

Strains or Sprains

Most back pain of the acute variety is caused by general strains or sprains. Strains occur when a muscle or tendon gets torn, and sprains happen when someone tears or over-stretches a ligament.

These can both happen from lifting something wrongly, twisting too suddenly, trying to lift something that is too heavy for your strength level, or simply stretching your back too far. These types of motions can also lead to back muscle spasms which are painful, too.

Ruptured or Herniated Discs

These occur when the discs get compressed and end up herniating (bulging out) or rupturing, leading to pain in the back that is often intense.

Radiculopathy

This is an issue that is the result of compression, injury, or inflammation of the nerve root in the spine. Numbness, pain, or tingling may result from pressure on the root of the spine, traveling or radiating to various other parts of the body that are connected with the nerve. This may also occur when a ruptured or herniated disc presses against the root or from spinal stenosis.

Sciatica

This is a type of radiculopathy which happens when the sciatic nerve (a big nerve that runs through the backside and reaches down the backs of your legs) becomes compressed. The compression leads to a burning or shock-like pain in the lower back, in addition to pain experienced down the length of one leg and the buttocks, often extending all the way down to the foot.

In severe cases of sciatica, muscle weakness and numbness may result in the leg of the sufferer. This happens when the signaling between nerves gets interrupted due to the nerve being pinched between the bone and disc. This condition can also result from a cyst or tumor that presses against the roots of the sciatic nerve or the nerve itself.

Spinal Stenosis

This refers to your spinal column getting narrower, which places pressure on the nerves and spinal cord, causing numbness or pain when you walk or do any other physical activity. Over the course of time, this can even lead to loss of the senses or weakness in the legs.

Injuries and Trauma

Injuries that occur from car accidents, falling, or playing sports can hurt your muscles, ligaments, or tendons and end up resulting in pain of the back. Traumatic injuries can cause your spine to compress too much, leading to ruptures or herniation of the intervertebral disc. This causes pressure to be placed on nerves attached to the spine. When nerves in the spine become irritated or compressed, it often ends up resulting in issues and pain or even sciatica.

Irregularities in the Spine

This can mean scoliosis (an unnatural curvature of your spinal column), which typically doesn't cause issues until later in life, general congenital irregularities in the spinal column, or lordosis, which refers to an arch in the back that is accentuated abnormally.

Pain in the lower back is not often related to a serious condition that is underlying, but when it is, you need to see a doctor right away.

7 - Serious Underlying Conditions Possibly Causing Back Pain

Tumors

These are quite a rare underlying cause of pain in the back. They can start in the back on rare occasions, but if they do appear in this area, it's typically from cancer that started in a different body part.

Infections in Parts of the Back

These are another rare cause of pain in the back. Infections in your back can lead to serious pain when they spread to the vertebra, intervertebral discs, or the joints that connect the pelvis to the lower part of the spine.

Kidney Stones

Kidney stones are an example of an underlying cause of back pain in some people. These are a very painful affliction that causes sharp discomfort, typically in the lower part of the back and on one side of the body only.

Aortic Aneurysms

These can cause back pain when they happen in the abdomen. This occurs when the blood vessel responsible for delivering blood to the legs, pelvis, and abdomen gets larger than it should. Pain in the back is typically a sign of this unnatural growth and means that a rupture may happen and should be prevented as soon as possible.

Osteoporosis

This is a metabolic disease of the bones which occurs when the bones gradually decrease in strength and density. This causes people to suffer breaks more easily, including vertebra fractures, leading to back pain oftentimes.

Fibromyalgia

Fatigue and muscle pain are two symptoms of this disease, which is known to be characterized by chronic pain. This can result in mild to severe back pain for sufferers.

Endometriosis

This ailment, which occurs when uterine tissue builds up outside of where it's supposed to (the uterus) and causes pain.

Inflammatory Joint Diseases

Rheumatoid arthritis, osteoarthritis, and general arthritis can contribute to pain in the lower back. Spondylitis, which is when the vertebra becomes inflamed, can also contribute to pain in the lower back.

No matter what the cause of the severity of the issue of back pain, everyone can agree that it's better to live without it. Thankfully, the better we understand the causes of this ailment, the better we can fix it. For certain cases, medical attention may be required, but there is plenty of work you can do at home to ease the process, which we will cover in this guide. We will also cover whether medical attention is necessary or not.

8 - Back Pain Development Risk Factors

Since serious back pain is one the most debilitating problems a person can face, you should do everything in your power to prevent getting to this level. What is it that causes some people to suffer from back pain while others never experience it, even mildly? In addition to the underlying issues we discussed in the previous chapters, there are some risk factors that can lead to this problem.

Fitness

People who do not make a point to exercise regularly are more likely to have back pain in their lives. When someone isn't fit physically, they have weaker abdominal and back muscles, which can't support their spine properly.

Some people are sedentary during the week, for example, those who work desk jobs, and try to get all their exercise in on the weekend. However, this presents a risk for back injuries, since the body isn't used to such motion. For this reason, everyone should make moderate exercise a part of their routine each and every day. Studies show that even low-intensity workouts will help keep the back healthy.

Age

People who are between 30 and 55 are likely to suffer their first back pain attack. Unfortunately, this tends to become even more common as time progresses from this age. As you age, your bones naturally weaken and can even develop fractures from osteoporosis. Simultaneously, your body's tone and the elasticity of your muscles decrease, causing the disks of your back to lose their flexibility and fluid. This means they can no longer cushion your vertebrae as they should. As you get older, your risk of developing a disorder called spinal stenosis goes up, as well.

Gaining Weight

Being obese or even semi-overweight, especially when it happens quickly, can lead to pain in the back because of the stress that gets placed upon your body. Maintaining a weight that is healthy for your size is necessary for preventing unnecessary pain and allowing your body to function as it should be able to.

Becoming Pregnant

Changes in the pelvis along with weight alterations can cause pregnant women to experience back pain, although it only lasts throughout the pregnancy, usually and returns to normal afterward.

Risks Involved with Occupation

Any career that involves pulling, pushing, or of course, heavy lifting, can result in back pain or other injuries. This is especially true when the job requires any twisting of the body or spine vibrating. Make sure you are learning the proper form for lifting and pulling if you have a job like this.

On the other side of the equation, there are jobs which are highly inactive that can lead to pain in the back, like jobs that require you to sit all day. Poor posture or not getting up often enough during the work day will often lead to pain the back. Make sure if you have a job that requires sitting, you do so in a chair with proper support and make sure to stand and shift position plenty of times throughout the day.

Genes

Certain issues resulting from genes, such as a special brand of spondylitis (an arthritis type that leads to the joints of the spine fusing together and reducing mobility) can cause people to suffer from back pain.

Mental Health

People wouldn't typically think of a connection between mental health and back pain, but it turns out that existing issues of mental health, such as depression or anxiety, can heavily influence the way someone perceives their back pain. Increased focus on this pain will make it seem more severe or overwhelming. When pain becomes chronic, it has a high tendency to increase mental health issues. In addition to this, stress can lead to tension of the muscles which results in pain for some.

Overloaded Backpacks for Kids

Pain in the back that doesn't happen as a result of injuries is not typical in kids, but a backpack that is too heavy can cause the muscles in the back to experience strain and fatigue. A backpack should never weigh more than 20% of the weight of the child to prevent this from happening.

How can you Prevent Back Pain?

Pain in the back that continues to recur from using the body improperly can be prevented by making sure you have correct posture, avoid motions that strain or jolt your back, and adopt the correct posture for lifting heavy items.

Keeping these Common Causes in Mind

Sometimes, helping your back heal or preventing future injuries can be as simple as staying aware of the risks involved. Many times, these issues come about in the first place because we aren't paying quite enough attention to what we are doing.

A lot of injuries resulting from work happen because of stressors like lifting heavy items, stress on the back from contact (which occurs when there is constant or repeated contact between the body and a sharp or hard object), awkward postures, vibrations from machinery, or repetitive movements.

Using Proper Furniture or Equipment

Equipment and furniture that has been designed ergonomically can help protect your back and body from injuries at work and home. Considering the future medical bills you could be avoiding by investing in this, it's a worthy item to spend money on, even if it costs a bit more than alternative options for the same products.

Consider Lumbar Supports to Help with Back Pain

Support to your abdominal region and lower back can be given by lumbar supports, which are elastic bands designed to be wide enough to cover these regions. The bands can be tightened and adjusted according to your body type and needs. Although these items have less evidence than other similar products as far as the support they provide, they are still used widely and work for some people. The best way to find out whether these are appropriate for you is to try them out yourself.

9 - Where to Begin with Treating Back Pain

In order to find out where you fall on the scale in terms of back pain severity and what to do about it, it's important to understand how professionals tend to treat this issue. No one wants to go to the doctor if it can be prevented because it's often expensive and time-consuming. Taking into consideration the steps a doctor will follow when examining you will help you decide whether that is necessary or not. So, how do you find out whether medical attention is needed?

Information on Back Pain Diagnostics

When someone goes to visit a doctor for issues related to the back, the doctor will look at the following considerations:

Pre-existing Conditions

Typically, a complete physical exam and observation of medical history are done to help identify existing conditions that could be contributing to your back pain. Any health issue that could be related will be covered.

Severity and Location of the Pain

While examining you, the health professional will question you about the site, onset, and intensity of the back pain you are experiencing. They will question you about how long the pain has been there and whether it inhibits your movements in any way.

Neurological Tests

In addition to an examination of the back, a neurological test will often be done to find out what is causing the pain and the best way to go about treating it. Keep in mind that the causes of pain in the lower back are often hard to determine, in spite of these examinations.

The Doctor may use Imaging Tests while Examining you. These types of tests are not always necessary, but for some they might be, in order to rule out spinal stenosis or tumors that could be causing pain.

X-Rays

While being examined for back pain causes, an x-ray might be conducted, with the intention of discovering any injured bones or vertebra. This test will show any fractures or misalignment in the vertebrae, along with other details in the structures of bone in the area. Issues in the discs of the back, ligaments, or muscles will not be visible on these imaging tests.

MRI tests (Magnetic Resonance Imaging)

This test results in a computer generated picture created from a magnetic force. While x-rays can only show details of structures of bone, MRIs will show details in the tendons, ligaments, blood vessels, and muscles.

This test might be necessary if you are suspected to have a ruptured or herniated disc, infection, a tumor, pressure on one of your nerves, or various inflammations. An MRI scan is a noninvasive method for determining conditions that need surgery, but are not usually necessary unless the medical history of the patient calls for it, or when the pain in the back is a recent occurrence.

Ultrasounds

This type of imagining, also known as sonography or ultrasound imagining or scanning, utilizes sound waves of high frequency to show pictures inside of the patient's body. The echoes of these sound waves are both recorded and shown as a visual picture in real time. This type of imagining can display tears in tendons, ligaments, muscles, or any other masses of tissue in a person's back.

Bone Scan Imaging

These types of scans can be used to monitor and detect disorders, fractures, or infections in the bone of the patient. The images generated from these scanners will be used to determine specific parts of the body that have irregular blood flow or abnormal metabolism in the bones. The images can also show whether there is any disease in your joints.

Self-Healing and Treatment for Back Pan

The information above is useful for people who are suffering severe or consistent pain, but for the rest of you, that may not be necessary. Depending on how severe your pain is, it's always preferred to attempt to heal yourself before consulting a professional. We have discussed the importance of physical fitness in treating and preventing back pain, which leads to the next question.

How are you Supposed to Exercise with Back Pain?

You may be wondering how it's possible to stay fit without intensifying the pain in your back. A lot of people will be surprised to find out that specific types of exercise actually reduce this pain. Some exercises that will be given in this guide can give you significant and quick pain relief, which will help you recover faster.

As soon as the pain disappears or decreases, other specific exercises can aid you in restoring the movement to your back and also strengthen your core muscles. Not only will this help you recover fully, but it will go a long way in preventing future injuries and pain in the back.

How are you to Know when Pain during Physical Activity is Something to Worry about? Many health care professionals believe that back pain increasing during physical activity is nothing to worry about, as long as it doesn't continue to increase after the exercise. This means that you should try to stay as active as you can.

An Intense Increase in Pain should be Examined

While some continuous pain during exercise is okay and nothing to worry about, if you notice a significant increase during physical fitness, you should stop immediately and notify your doctor.

Keep in mind that this book is intended to be a general guide and that not everything in the book is suited for everyone. If you have any doubts at all on whether or not something in this guide is appropriate for you and your specific situation, consult your doctor.

How to Choose Exercises to Avoid an Increase in Back Pain

It is of utmost importance to know how to select your exercises in order to avoid worsening the issue. You can start by knowing how to determine whether your back condition is worsening. One way to know is if you notice:

Spreading Symptoms

Your back may be getting worse if the pain and symptoms are spreading lower into the buttocks, away from the middle of your back, or into one or both of your legs.

This Warning Sign can Happen in the Following Ways

This could occur in certain standing or sitting positions as well as during activity or exercise of any kind. It's a sign that the condition is worsening. Instead of that, what should you be aiming for?

The Goal here should be "Pain Centralization"

The positive aspect with this effect from exercise is that you can also experience the opposite of spreading symptoms, meaning that the symptoms move away from your buttock or legs and toward the center of the back. This is the ultimate goal of any exercise used to lessen back pain and is a great sign. It means that you are getting better and working your way toward full recovery. It's perfectly possible to find positions and exercises that cause this to happen. As soon as the pain and symptoms have made their way to the middle of your back, or "centralized", they typically get better and go away altogether with continued fitness regimes.

10 - Exercises that Work Best for Centralizing Back Pain

There are four main exercises to do, which are commonly most effective for reducing back pain symptoms. These are:

Pushups (or Press-ups)

Standard pushups can be a great way to stretch out as well as strengthen your back. Of course, if the pain is too severe to get into this position it should be avoided. If your body is not used to doing this exercise, you can start doing easier pushups by balancing on your knees instead of feet.

Walks on Level and Solid Ground

Going on frequent walks can do a lot to help with easing back pain. Make sure you are wearing shoes that have adequate and proper support and that you are walking on level ground instead of rough terrain. This will get your blood flowing and do a lot to stretch out your lower back, easing the pain gradually.

Backbends while Standing up

This is an activity that should be done very gently and

gradually, especially if you suffer from severe pain. Only bend as far back as you can stand without increasing your pain substantially. This intensity can be adjusted over time as you acclimate to this motion.

When you are partaking in these fitness activities, along with other exercises, always pay attention to the level of your pain. It should be going away, centralizing, or staying at the same level. If it seems to be worsening, this is a warning sign.

11 - The Importance of Posture when it comes to Back Issues

One of the most important factors for your back is the quality of your posture. In addition to exercise, adopting appropriate posture is essential to healing yourself, whether you are sitting or standing.

Posture while Seated

When you are sitting, try not to sit for longer than you absolute have to, and avoid slouching at all costs. If you notice that your back pain symptoms are worsening while you sit, or moving downward toward the legs or buttocks, check the way you are sitting. For a lot of back pain sufferers, sitting up straight could help to lessen and centralize symptoms.

Posture is Part of your Fitness Regimen

You may find it helpful to think of sitting up straight as part of your fitness regimen and an exercise to increase the stamina of your muscles and build better habits of sitting. When you heal yourself of your pain, sitting up straight will often keep pain from coming back.

If you have to Sit for Long Periods

Sometimes, sitting for long periods of time may be unavoidable. In this case, you may find it helpful to place a support behind the back to keep it properly aligned, with its natural curve being deepened by the support. You should also try to keep your hips raised slightly above the height of your knees.

12 - How to Exercise once your Pain has Abated

In a lot of cases, you might improve or even entirely eliminate pain within a day or two. As soon as the pain is improved or gone altogether:

Work your Way Up Slowly

You can carefully and gradually improve and increase the range of your body's motion, beginning with simple exercises that involve bending forward.

Keep Going

As long as the pain does not come back, worsen, or start spreading to other parts of the body, you should continue your exercise and also remember to maintain correct posture. Many people find that this does a lot to keep back pain away.

13 - The Importance of Strength Training Exercises

A lot of people who experience pain in the back have weak muscles in the core of their bodies. Focusing on strength training will help you prevent future pain and issues in your back. This is one of the most valuable activities you can partake in for your health, overall. All postures and movements of the body (sitting up straight included) require adequate flexibility and strength of the muscles. This means you need to do some stretching as well as strength training. Strengthening your lower back is important because it:

Helps Repair Injuries

This happens as a result of increased blood flow in the body. Injuries can only be repaired if they receive adequate nutrients, and increased blood flow helps with this delivery process. The muscles you are exercising will receive nutrients due to the increased blood flow, along with tissues neighboring the muscles.

While aerobic fitness activities have this effect as well (biking, swimming, or walking for example), strength training is especially effective.

Improves Stamina and Strength

The overall function of your body in day to day life will be helped with this. Working on strengthening your muscles, in general, will help you function more easily in life. Remember that, while strengthening your back, your leg muscles, and core need to be focused on, as well. This is because these muscles give your body the stability it needs in the core and back to improve your overall gait and balance.

Since this will help you perform your daily tasks with better stamina and ease, you will be less likely to hurt yourself or take a spill. While gyms or certain fitness equipment can help, there are plenty of inexpensive and low-tech methods for strengthening your muscles yourself, at home. The added benefit of going this route is that you can start today instead of waiting.

Quality care of your lack should include exercises centered around pain relief along with correct stretching motions, as well as moderate strength training exercises and activities. Attempting to heal yourself with these methods will help you make a good recovery and also help you with preventing problems in the future.

14 - Where should you Start with Back Pain Exercises?

Extensions from a Standing Posture

To do this exercise, begin with your hands placed so that your fingers are touching the center of your lower back. Bend your body back as far as you can without straining yourself or worsening your pain, as you press inward with your hands. Hold this posture for a couple of seconds and repeat this motion up to 10 times. Each time you adopt this posture, try to bend a bit further. If you don't experience a worsening of your back pain symptoms, repeat this exercise once every couple of hours.

Walking

When you are starting out with introducing walking into your routine, start with 10 minutes per day and gradually increase until you are at 30 minutes or more. This distance and time should be adjusted according to your preference and tolerance. Only walk as fast or as far as is suited for your specific situation and pain level.

The Posture of Standing Exercise

For this position, draw your head backwards, letting your chin tuck in and fall. Your shoulders and ears should be aligned vertically with your hips and in balance with the position of your legs.

Facing Downward on your Elbows

Lift your body up using your elbows, allowing the lower part of your back to sag downward. Hold this position for 15 seconds and repeat the motion 4 times. Do this every couple of hours, as long as your symptoms and pain do not worsen.

Pushups (or Press-ups)

For this exercise, press upward using your arms, allowing the lower part of your back to hang loosely. Hold this position for a couple of seconds before resuming the lying pose. Repeat this motion up to 10 times, allowing your lower back to sag lower with each repetition. If the pain worsens, stop immediately. As long as it is comfortable to do so, repeat this exercise every couple of hours.

The Sitting Position for Back Pain

Your shoulders and ears must be level over your hips, resulting in a similar lower back hollow as you have while standing in an erect posture.

If you start doing these exercises faithfully each day, you should notice a quick improvement to the state of your back. Always remember that if your pain starts getting worse, you should stop immediately or at least pause to take frequent breaks and go easier. We will cover a few more exercises later on in this book.

15 - Treatment Information and Options for Curing Back Pain

How back pain will go about getting treated typically depends on the type of pain, meaning whether it is a chronic or acute pain. Generally, a health care provider will recommend surgery only in the case of nerve damage that continues to worsen, or when medical tests prove that corrective surgery is needed for changings in the structure of the back. The most commonly used treatments for back pain are:

Movement and Activity

Contrary to what some may believe, resting in bed should be done sparingly. People with back pain should start a routine for stretching and resume their ordinary daily schedules as soon as they can, as long as they avoid motions that make their pain worse.

There has been plenty of evidence that proves that people who refrain from bed rest and continue their typical activities after their back pain starts seem to have better flexibility in their backs than people who rested for a week in bed. Other medical evidence has suggested that resting in bed alone could make pain in the back worse and even lead to extra issues like depression, blood clots, and deteriorating muscle tone.

Cold or Hot Packs

Although this method hasn't been proven definitively to resolve back pain quickly, they do help tremendously with reducing inflammation and easing pain with chronic, sub-acute, or acute pain. This method also allows sufferers of back pain to engage in a wider range of mobility.

Strength Training

These types of exercises are not recommended for lower back pain that is acute, but is more effective as a way to help the recovery along from sub-acute or chronic pain in the lower back.

For people who suffer from back pain as a result of irregularities of the skeletal system, strength training, and maintaining muscle is especially important. Medical professionals can give you more information on which specific exercises are best suited for your ailment and improving posture, coordination, and muscle strength, if necessary. Evidence has shown promise for yoga greatly improving chronic pain in the back.

Physical Therapy

These types of programs are highly beneficial and are designed to strengthen central groups of muscle that support your spinal column, overall back, help with flexibility and mobility, and aid you in proper posture and positioning. These programs are typically used in conjunction with other treatments and interventions.

Medications for Back Pain Sufferers

In some cases, medication may be necessary for back pain, though this is something only a professional health care provider can tell you for certain. A large range of medicines is available for treating chronic and acute back pain. While there are some you can get over the counter, stronger ones require a prescription from a doctor:

OTC

Medications that are available over the counter, such as aspirin or acetaminophen can help a lot with back pain, especially milder or temporary symptoms.

Opioid Medications

For more serious pain and symptoms, you may get prescribed an opioid medication such as hydrocodone, codeine, or morphine. These medications should never be used unless they were prescribed by a health care professional, and should only be used for short periods of time since they are highly addictive.

There is some controversy about the effectiveness of these types of medications since these drugs can lead to and worsen depression symptoms, which adds to pain in the back. This should be kept in mind while making decisions on whether or not to go on opioid pain medications for back pain.

Anti-irritant Medications

Medications that have been developed to counter irritations, such as topical sprays or creams, can stimulate your skin's nerves to cause feelings of cold or warmth, intended to help dull pain symptoms. These topical formulas can stimulate your flow of blood in the skin and also work to get rid of or reduce inflammation.

16 - When Medication is not Enough to Cure your Symptoms

Acupuncture Therapy

This is a method that has been shown to have moderate effectiveness for people who suffer from back pain in a chronic or severe way. What this involves is the insertion of needles into specific parts of your body. While some practitioners claim a metaphysical explanation of this that states that the process is clearing away your body's life force blockages, others believe that the stimulation caused by the needles releases chemicals with natural pain killing properties.

Empirical evidence on the effectiveness of acupuncture is still needed, but many people claim that it helps, which makes it worth a try for people suffering from serious pain.

Surgery for Back Pain

This is obviously an option that most people would like to avoid at all costs. However, when all other attempts at curing back pain fail, it may be the best choice. While some options for surgery have effects that are almost immediate, others take a few months to go into full effect. Only you, along with your health care provider, can make an informed decision on whether surgery is right for you.

17 - General Tips for Avoiding Back Pain

In an ideal world, back pain wouldn't even exist for us. When it's too late and you have already suffered from back pain, you would probably like to do everything in your power to avoid going through it again. So what are some general ways to avoid back pain from ever occurring or re-occurring? Here are several recommendations for a healthy and pain-free back.

Low-Impact Fitness

After any period of time where you have been sedentary (inactive), you should engage in a routine of simple and gentle exercises. This can be anything from stationary bike riding to swimming, to power walking for 30 minutes a day. These simple activities will improve the flexibility and overall strength of your muscles.

Yoga for Preventing Back Issues

Yoga also does a lot to help with strengthening and stretching of the muscles of the body and the general quality of your body's posture. Contact a health care professional to find a list of exercises that are low impact and appropriate for your age group, specifically designed for strengthening your core muscles and back.

Stretching before Fitness

Making sure your body is sufficiently warmed up before engaging in any physical activity or strenuous movements will reduce the risk of harming your back because your muscles will be prepared for the motions.

Break the Slouching Habit

Always make sure you sit up straight whether you are sitting down or standing up. Your lower back supports your weight a lot easier when there is less curvature going on, meaning that you should always have your weight as balanced as possible on both feet, any time you are standing up.

Choosing the Correct Chairs

Make sure you sit in chairs that are equipped with proper lumbar support, along with the proper height and position for sitting. While you're sitting, especially for long periods of time, keep your shoulders pinned back. When you have to sit for long periods, make sure you shift positions frequently and get up to stretch your legs and walk periodically to prevent the buildup of tension in your muscles.

Placing a pillow in the curve of your lower back can help with support, as well as elevating your feet during long periods of time that you have to sit.

Having Work Surfaces of Proper Height

Take into account the surfaces that you are working with, whether it be a desk at work or the kitchen counter at home, and be sure that they are a comfortable height for you to reduce slouching or reaching, which can play a toll on your back after prolonged periods of time.

Sleeping Postures for Preventing Back Pain

People who sleep on their side with their knees up tend to have less pain in their back, since this position helps reduce the spine's curvature, get rid of pressure, and open up the spine's joints. You should also try to sleep on firmer mattresses when possible.

Selecting the Right Shoes

Shoes with the proper support go a long way in protecting your body against back pain. This means shoes that are comfortable to walk in and ideally have lower heels. If you have to wear high heels, since they shift the center of your body's gravity and can put unnecessary strain on the lower part of your back, only wear them for limited periods of time, bringing lower heeled shoes to switch to when possible.

Proper Lifting Form and Guidelines

You should never attempt to lift items that are overly heavy for your strength or body. When you do lift, do so using your knees, with your back straightened, head down, and pulling in your stomach muscles. Try to hold the heavy items as close to your body as you can and never twist as you lift.

When possible, you should always try to push heavy objects, rather than pulling them, since this is less likely to injure your back or other parts of the body.

Stay a Healthy Weight

Nutrition is important in many aspects of life, and back pain is no exception. Making sure you are receiving the proper nutrition will keep you from gaining excessive amounts of weight around the middle of your body, which will eventually wreak havoc on the muscles of your lower back. Making sure you get enough vitamin D, phosphorus, and calcium will ensure that you are taking care of your bones, which will do even more to prevent back pain.

Stop Smoking

In case you needed an extra reason to get rid of this bad habit, now you have one. Smoking decreases the flow of blood to the lower part of your spine, meaning that it contributes to the degeneration of your back's discs. Engaging in the habit of smoking also means you are increasing your risk for getting osteoporosis, and also lessening the healing abilities of your body, in general. In addition to this, coughing, which can result from smoking a lot, may cause you to suffer from back pain.

Wear less Tight Clothes

Tight clothes have a tendency to interfere with sitting, walking, and bending, which can worsen or cause back pain. You should be especially wary of jeans that are very tight.

Be Picky about your Briefcase or Bag

When you are selecting the briefcase or bag you will use, try to pick one with an adjustable, wide strap that you can place diagonally over your body, since the weight will be more evenly distributed this way. Try to switch shoulders periodically. In addition to this, if you have a bag that won't reach over your head in this way, shift which hand you use to carry it every so often.

A lot of people carry around stuff that they don't actually need. Whenever possible, only carry light backpacks or purses to prevent straining your back more than you absolutely need to.

Get a Lighter Wallet

Sitting down on a wallet that has too much in it can contribute to pain in your back. If you have to sit for long periods of time, at work or while driving, remove the wallet from your pants to create a more even sitting surface.

Pay Close Attention to your Body

When it comes down to it, we're all built differently. This means that what causes or helps back pain in one person may differ completely for another. You should always pay close attention to what your body is telling you in order to know what works for you when it comes to preventing or helping your back.

Get rid of your Back Brace

When you are suffering from pain in your back, you may be tempted to baby the muscles, but professionals state that back braces should not be used or, at least, used very rarely. Although they are helpful when it comes to certain activities, like lifting heavy objects, you shouldn't wear them for longer than 15 minutes. Wearing these devices for long periods of time, such as an entire work day, causes your muscles to grow dependent on the device.

Your muscles are intended to create stability for your core, back, and upper body as a whole and relying on back braces means that your muscles get weaker.

Consult a Professional

Seeing a doctor is not always necessary. After all, there is plenty you can do to heal yourself from the comfort of your own home using the information in this book. However, some people may need some extra help in addition to what they can do on their own. Coming up with a fitness plan that is individually tailored to your needs is a must for managing any kind of back pain, but there is no specific regimen, activity plan, or medicine that works for everyone. This is where consulting a professional can come in handy.

Some people may require more strengthening in their core, while others might just need more flexibility and stretching. Talking to a chiropractor or physical therapist with expertise in the area of back pain and care will help you find the perfect solution for you.

Consider Trying Different Therapy Options

This can mean either official or non-official therapy. Back

pain, as mentioned earlier in this book, often goes hand in hand with anxiety, depression, or other mental health issues. This is because your state of mind and mood has a direct result on the way you perceive and experience pain.

Talking to a therapist or even a sympathetic friend can go a long way in helping you heal yourself, by lightening the emotional burden of the situation. You will also receive the benefit of a fresh perspective on your situation which can help the way you perceive and experience the pain.

Utilize Techniques for General Relaxation

Studies have proven that engaging in relaxing activities like deep breathing, yoga, and meditation that ease the mind in general can have an amazing impact on your back. If you learn how to consciously relax, you can also consciously control the way you perceive the pain level in your back.

Consult the Higher Ups at your Place of Work

Since so many instances of back pain are caused by job

factors, you should speak with the HR department at your workplace or your boss. This could help you with finding a solution using adjustments to your work environment.

18 - More Simple Exercises to Help

As mentioned a few different times in this guide, exercise is one of the most surefire ways to aid you in managing and preventing back pain in your life. The specific type of fitness activity you engage in matters less than the fact that you are engaging in plenty of movement and staying active. While some believe that swimming is the most beneficial, others prefer to do yoga, while others still like running or walking better. What is important in the choice you make is that you enjoy the activity you're doing. This will make you much more likely to stick with it long enough to enjoy the benefits that come along with it. There are a number of exercises you should try to help heal your back.

Swimming Regularly

Swimming is the lowest impact exercise you can engage in since the water takes the strain off of all of your muscles and joints. Some also claim that swimming is the most thorough workout you can engage in since it works every part of your body.

Getting into Pilates for your Back

Pilates is great for this since it strengthens your spine and muscles, promoting erect and quality posture for sitting, standing, and walking.

General Programs for Fitness

Any fitness regimen that involves cardiovascular exercise and includes the muscles of your core and back will go a long way in helping you heal your back. This can be anything from a dance program, to martial arts, to sports.

Specific Exercises to Help Back Pain

Not only do these exercises stretch out your back to help protect it against injuries, but they can help ease existing pain as well. Following a routine, with each of these exercises, each day will help your pain a lot, especially if you stay faithful to it. The great news about these exercises is that they don't require any equipment, so you can begin today.

A Morning Warm up

Stand up straight, placing your feet apart slightly, with your arms held out in front of you or in front of the chest, folded.

Slightly bend the knees and also bend the hips so that your back is parallel to the ground below and flat, curving your lower back so that your bottom is sticking out.

Exhale as you go down, inhaling as you go back up. Repeat this exercise up to 12 times.

The Partial Squat Exercise

Stand in an erect posture, holding your arms in front of the chest, folded and your feet a natural width apart.

Slightly bend the knees, bringing your thighs about halfway parallel to the ground below, then resume the original position.

Move on to placing your thighs about parallel with the ground below (a half squatting position), but don't go deeper than this.

Exhale as you go down, inhaling as you go back up. Repeat this exercise five times, if possible, making your way up to 10 gradually.

Leg and Arm Raise Exercise

Go down to the floor with your body on all fours, with your hands on the ground level with your shoulders and the knees apart slightly. Your thighs and arms should be in a vertical position.

The Cat-Cow Yoga Position

This pose is great for stretching out your back and abdomen muscles. On all fours, arch your back while looking down at the ground below you.

Now, lower your stomach so that it's dipping toward the ground, then hollow your back as you look upward. Repeat this up to 10 times each session. This position may not be suitable for pregnant women.

The Arm Swinging Exercise

Get on all fours onto the ground, raising one hand from the

floor and reach down under your body, stretching as far as possible.

For the second part of this exercise, swing your arm outward, from the side of your body, as far as it will reach, returning after to the beginning position.

Keep your eyes on the hand that is moving, alternating hands each time. Do this in repetitions of 10.

The Side Raise with Bent Leg Exercise

Place yourself on the ground, down on all fours, swinging your leg, while bending it, from the hip and to the side, returning it afterward to center.

Do this 10 more times and then switch to the other leg.

The Back Arching Fitness Position

Lie down on the floor, facing down, then push your body up using your arms, with the hands level with the shoulders.

Make sure your pelvis stays on the ground and raise the back from the ground, repeating this motion up to 10 times for each set.

Knee Raisers

Go down onto all fours, drawing each knee up to the elbow opposite of the knee, alternating each time.

Go back to the position you held originally, and repeat this 10 times per leg.

The Trunk Rotation Exercise

Sit on the ground with your legs crossed, then twist the shoulders to the side, putting your hand on the ground behind your body.

Put your other arm outside of the opposite knee, twisting your body toward the opposite knee and holding the position for a few seconds. Use your arm as a way to push against your knee, and repeat this up to five times for each side of your body.

The Rowing Upright Position

Stand up straight, placing your feet level with your hips, and your arms down at the sides of your body. Then bring both hands up right below the chin.

Simultaneously, bring the elbows upward as far as you can, to your head. Then, put your arms back down at the sides of your body.

Inhale on your way upward, and exhale as you go back down. Repeat these motions 10 times for each set.

Simple Chest and Knee Combination Exercise

For this exercise, pull your knee up toward your chest, pulling gently and holding the position for 10 seconds at a time. Do this four times for each leg.

This can be done with a single knee at a time or both simultaneously, as you see fit.

Extensions Face Down on the Floor

Put your hands behind your back, while lying face down on the ground. Then lift your shoulders and head off of the ground, holding the position for five seconds at a time.

Repeat this motion three times for each set.

Arm and Leg Straightening Exercise

For this routine, get down on all fours, then reach your arm outward, straightening the opposite leg behind your body. You can tighten your abdominal muscles in order to make this easier, then hold the position for up to 10 seconds.

Gently go back to the position you started at, then alternate the arm and leg you do this with, repeating each side five times.

19 - More Causes and How to Prevent Them

For a lot of people out there, back pain seems inevitable, like a fact of life, they have no choice but to live with. However, we have more control over this than we might believe. It's possible to hurt your back in many different ways, but there are a few specific causes that are most common and prevalent. These include never stretching your body enough, not being conscious of the way you move your body, and general wear and tear on the back from years of use. There are number of common bad habits that hurt the back and we will explore what to do about them.

Reckless Weekend Behavior

Too often, people hurt themselves playing sports on the weekend, because they overestimate their own strength or flexibility. The problem is that so many people life sedentary lifestyles during the week and then think that they can perform like athletes without training. This causes pain in the back and oftentimes, injuries.

This doesn't just apply to sports. Even simple activities like your weekend to-do list can be harmful if your body was idle the entire week prior to that. This can mean bending over your garden, cleaning the house, or standing at your work-bench all day. The solution to this issue is making sure that you don't reserve your physical activity for specific days but try to introduce plenty of exercise and movement into every day of your life, focusing heavily on getting a stronger and more flexible core. Your side abdominal muscles are especially important when it comes to preventing injuries in your back.

Bad Techniques for Lifting Heavy Items

People think that just because they are strong enough to lift heavy items, that's all they need to do it right. This is a mistaken belief that leads to many easily preventable back woes. Be sure to engage your abdominal muscles while you lift to give your back the support it needs and keep it pain-free.

Bend at the knees, never the waist, while lifting. Remember that the further an object is away from your body, the worse it is for your back. Don't ever hold an object below your knees or above your armpit. Never move an item that is heavier than 20% of what you yourself weigh.

Not Paying Attention to your Body throughout the Day

Simple household chores, even ones as easy as doing dishes or taking the trash out can have a negative impact on your spine if you don't use your body often or pay attention to the way you are moving. People make the mistake of assuming that only jerky motions or heavy lifting can hurt your back, but you can just as easily injure yourself doing something simple.

If you aren't paying attention to the motions of your body and instead are operating on "auto-pilot" mode, this could lead to issues. People tend to get hurt more often at work when they are about to be done for the day since they start losing focus and get fatigued mentally. You can prevent this hazard by keeping the muscles of your core active and engaged throughout the day, and by focusing in general on your physical movements.

You can do this in a simple and easy way by pulling your belly button back toward the spinal column and envision yourself in a corset that is pulling the abs in from the sides. If you do this repeatedly throughout your day, as you go through your typical activities, particularly while bending your body or lifting objects, you will have better support for the back and gradually build strength, as well.

Sitting at a Desk or in a Car for Long Periods

In our modern world, people sit far too often. You sit while you drive to work while watching your favorite shows on television, and some of you even sit all day while at work. It turns out that this is horrible for your back and leads to issues, but why is that?

We simply aren't built for sitting around. We evolved to walk and be in motion often. The discs of your back have a spongy texture to them, intended to provide a cushion for your spine's vertebrae, but they don't naturally have a quality supply of blood. When you engage in plenty of motion, fluid can circulate throughout these discs. If your body is still all day, the fluid runs out, meaning that your discs aren't getting the nutrition they need to do their job.

Living in front of a computer or spending a lot of time driving will wear out these discs, leading to extra stress for the back and extra risk for injuries. Keep in mind that the discs of your back need motion to stay nourished and do what they are meant to do. Sitting for long periods is bad for your neck and back and leads to damage that can be permanent or long-lasting. In fact, research has proven that sitting down actually places, even more, pressure on the spine than standing or lying down.

But the worst sitting posture you can adopt involves leaning forward while sitting. What happens when you do this is that your pelvis locks up and your spine flexes, placing pressure on the discs at the forefront of your vertebrae. Arching forward and exaggerating your spine's natural curve puts, even more, pressure on these discs. This type of pressure will put you at a risk of rupturing a disk.

20 - When you Must Sit for Long Periods, do This to Help with Back Issues:

Every 20 Minutes, Get Up

This may not be possible for long drives, but try to walk around a bit at least once every 20 minutes or half hour at the most. You can set a timer or screen saver for your work computer in order to remember to do this.

Start a habit where you go get some water every half hour, and when you have to pick up the phone at work, take this chance to shift positions and stand to stretch.

Eye Level Reading

When you have to sit and read for long periods, whether it be books or a computer screen at work, make sure your spine is aligned correctly by keeping your material for reading at the level of your eyes. Avoid bending over whenever possible, especially over your desk at work for long periods of time.

Remember that as often as is possible, you should keep your

spine held straight. This means selecting a quality chair for good support and adjusting it so your feet can stay on the ground flat. Remember to keep large items out of your back pockets since this interferes with the alignment of your spine, and place a rolled up towel at the small of the back if this helps your posture at work.

If None of this Helps your Back...

If you have severe pain that doesn't go away, you must consult a professional, since you could have a serious underlying issue. If you are suffering severe pain that doesn't go away within a full 48 hours, this is a sign that you should consult a doctor immediately. Remember that prevention is better than needing treatment, so always treat your back right and stay strong and flexible.

21 - How to Sleep Well with Back Pain

The average person spends at least a third of their life sleeping, so perhaps it will come as a surprise that so many of us don't see the connection from any pain or symptoms we may suffer related to back pain and the quality of our sleep. It's time to start paying attention to this connection to see if the way you sleep may be contributing to your pain problems.

The Cycle of Bad Sleep Patterns and Habits and Back Pain

If you suffer from back in the back, it doesn't go away when you lie down to go to sleep. Oftentimes problems with sleeping and back pain go hand in hand and fuel each other, creating a vicious cycle of issues. Back pain symptoms can make it hard, or even impossible, to get quality sleep. Sometimes, these symptoms even get worse as a direct result of not getting quality sleep. That being said, what is to be done about this problem? Fortunately, there are some simple changes you can make to help this issue.

Now you should consider the following tricks to get quality

sleep with back pain symptoms.

Regularly Re-evaluate your Mattress

If you tend to get better sleep when you stay overnight at hotels, wake up too often with pain in your lower back, and have a mattress that is getting worn out, you should think about re-vamping your bed. In fact, people should purchase new mattresses about every five years or so. Studies have suggested that the majority of people report significant back pain improvements when they switch to a new and improved mattress.

If you can afford to get a brand new mattress, try to test out a few choices before making your final decision. With how much of your life you spend sleeping, it's worth taking the time to make the best choice. Go to a bed store and lie down on some mattresses that look promising. Try to find a choice that keeps your spine in the same posture you have when you stand up straight. Mattresses that are firm or at least medium firm are typically the best for general spine and back health.

An Alternative to a New Mattress

For some people, going out and buying a new mattress is not possible, since they can be quite expensive. If that's the case for you, there's another option you can try. Put some plywood support slats between the base of your mattress and the mattress itself until you can afford to purchase a new, quality mattress.

Placing your Mattress on the Floor

Since having a firmer surface helps a lot with easing and preventing back pain, you could attempt to move your mattress to the ground to see if this helps. Of course, this can be just a temporary solution until you can buy a new mattress or new bed altogether. A lot of people find that they sleep much better and suffer far fewer issues with their back while sleeping on the ground instead of on a bed.

Homemade Sleep Supports to Try

When you are sleeping on your back, you can place a pillow or rolled up blanket underneath your knees. If you tend to sleep on your side, placing the support between the knees is effective for helping to prevent and ease back pain in the night.

Remember that the natural curve of your spine should be maintained whenever possible and that a lack of this often causes back pain. To keep this curve intact while you are lying in bed at night, try using a towel that has been rolled up and wrap it around your body at the waist, tied together at the front of your body.

Paying Attention to How you Get into and Out of your Bed

This is another typical activity we do countless times throughout our life, but probably never see in connection with the pain we experience in our back. To heal yourself, pay attention to this and:

Do not Jerk your Body Upward

For back pain sufferers, the pain can worsen a lot if they are too jerky with their movements while getting out of and into bed. When you are in a lying position, ease yourself up slowly.

Lying Down

When you are getting into bed, you should first sit on the edge of your mattress, holding your body up using your hands, bend your body at the knees, and gently lie down on the mattress onto the side of your body.

Getting Up

When you are getting out of bed in the morning or the middle of the night, first roll yourself into a side-lying position, bending your knees, and proceed to push your body up using your hands, simultaneously swinging your lower body off the edge of the mattress. Never bend yourself forward at the middle of your body, since this can lead to strain for your back.

More Tips for Sleeping with Back Pain

In addition to making sure you have the correct support and posture while lying in bed, along with getting into and out of bed correctly, you should also:

Preventing Resting for Too Long at a Time

Although rest can definitely help in healing, make sure you aren't lying in bed for multiple days at a time after you hurt yourself. Although it can be tempting to do this, it will often make the pain worse.

If you are experiencing pain that is so bad that you must lie down for relief, you should make sure to stand up every once in a while and move around to prevent more stiffness and symptoms. This will help you get better rest in the evenings when you go to sleep.

Try not to Eat too Much before Sleep

Eating huge meals right before you go to bed can lead to digestive issues and also lower qualities of sleep. Try to have dinner at least a couple of hours before lying down to go to bed at night.

Limit Alcohol and Caffeine

This is especially important at night since both of these substances can mess with the quality of your sleep.

If you follow all of the tips outlined in this chapter, there's a chance that you might still notice that your back pain worsens in the night, regardless of your attempts to make it better. If this is the case for you, you should definitely notify your doctor, since it could be signaling a deeper issue that requires attention.

Conclusion

Back pain can be one of the most debilitating afflictions imaginable, depending on its severity. Whether your pain is mild or severe, it takes away from your overall quality of life and should definitely be improved to the best of your abilities. I hope this book was able to help you to gain some insight as to what may be causing your back pain, how to improve it, and what to do to prevent future pain in your back.

Simple changes in habit can make a big difference in your susceptibility to injury. The next step is to figure out what lifestyle changes will help to prevent back pain in the future, so you can get on with living a fully functional life free from worry. Small changes each day in the right direction are of utmost importance.

Book 2: Sciatica

Pain Relief Guide (Exercises, Back Pain Relief, Natural Remedies, Home Treatment)

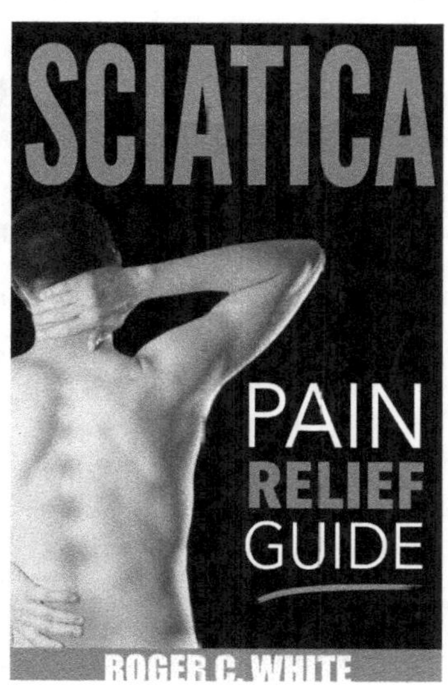

1 - Introduction

I would like to briefly congratulate you for purchasing this helpful guide for Sciatica: Pain Relief Guide: Exercise—Back Pain Relief—Natural Remedies & Home Treatment.

You can follow some of the steps provided to reduce the pain of sciatica nerve pain through exercises as well as through other methods. You will discover many new ways to bend and move your body to eliminate some of the pain of sciatica.

You will need to discover what works best for you. To ensure you aren't proceeding with a plan that could harm you in the long-term, it is recommended to have a full diagnosis from your physician.

You will discover it takes several professions to treat your sciatica pain, whether it is a chiropractor or a surgeon, or home remedies; you now have a plan.

It is time to be in charge of your life and live it to its fullest!

2 - Understanding Sciatica

What is Sciatica?

The medical term for sciatica is radiculopathy. The sciatic nerve is the largest nerve in your body which has two branches—the peroneal and the tibial nerve. The sciatica is the pain in the leg caused by a pinched nerve in your lower (lumbar) spine/back and is described by some as a shooting 'electricity' type of pain. Even though the pain begins in the nerve endings located on both sides of the lower spine, the pain also radiates through the sciatic nerve which is located on both legs from the butt to the foot.

The sciatic nerve passes between the gluteus maximus and gluteus medius (the deep buttock muscles), through the back of the thigh muscles, and down the outer edge of the leg to the foot.

Sciatica is considered a symptom which might feel like a shooting pain that can make sitting or standing difficult—or —it could feel like a severe leg cramp as the pain travels down your spine and your legs with a zipper effect. However, the pain can radiate from a mild ache to the jolt of pain similar to an electric shock.

A report in 2005 from the Journal of Neurosurgery: Spine estimated over 5% of the United States adult population suffers painful sciatica.

The Symptoms and How Long They Last

Five to ten percent of all patients who suffer from lower-back pain are suffering from sciatica. Many people can be relieved of the symptom within approximately six weeks, but for others, it could be longer. Other than the pain suffered in your back, you may also notice some of these symptoms:

- Tingling—an abnormal sensation—called (paresthesia)

- Pain from sitting which is accompanied by tingling sensations in the back of your thigh

- Numbness and weakness or the loss of feeling in the affected leg that can cause your knees to buckle when you stand from sitting

- Reduced reflexes in your knee and Achilles' tendon

- Difficulty exercising or moving

- Pain while sleeping

- Feel stiff

- Inflammation in the lower back or around your thighs after standing or sitting for a specified amount of time.

- Foot Drop: This condition will make you unable to flex your ankles enough to walk on your heels.

NOTE: If any of these symptoms are present seek immediate medical assistance:

1. Loss of bladder or bowel function

2. Severe weakness in the affected leg

3. Loss of feeling in the affected leg

Risk Factors involved with Sciatic Nerve Pain

Inflammation can cause injuries to take longer to heal, but

certain risk factors can intensify the problems including:

Stress

High levels of mental stress, fear, or other emotional issues can trigger tension and panic. These issues impact your musculature and posture which can trigger the sciatic nerve pain since it is usually the first body part to respond.

Tallness

Taller people are more susceptible to disc deterioration (research proven).

Age

Older age cause changes in the spine such as bone spurs or herniated discs.

Obesity

Being obese or overweight places additional stress on the spine.

Diabetes

The condition increases your nerve damage risk because of the way your body uses sugar.

Cigarette Smoking

You can help prevent disc degeneration if you avoid or stop smoking cigarettes. Nicotine can especially irritate the sciatic nerve.

Excessive Alcohol Usage

Alcohol can deplete your body of vital nutrients necessary for good bone health.

Prolonged Sitting

Individuals sitting for extended periods of time or have a sedentary lifestyle are more likely to develop sciatica versus active people.

Occupation

Working/driving with exposure to the vibration from a

vehicle for extended amounts of time or having a job which requires you to carry heavy loads or requires you to twist your back in the process can become a sciatica trigger.

Ambien Usage

Note: The insomnia drug has been linked to individuals as harmful and it has been linked to sciatica in some cases. It is best to consult your doctor for an alternative source of a sleeping aid.

Steps to Protect Your Back

Many of the problems which can lead to sciatica pain can be prevented. These are just a few of those ways:

Regular Exercise

A good exercise program can help to strengthen your back and abdomen to work toward better support for your spine.

Good Posture

Supporting our back with good posture can be practiced when you are standing, sitting, or sleeping. While sleeping, you can use a pillow under your knees or sleep on your side/back.

While sitting, use a swivel based chair with good back support and arm rests. Try placing a rolled towel or pillow in the small of your back to maintain the body's normal curve. Keep your hips and knees level.

This is the best standing posture pose:

1. Stand up completely straight with your ears in alignment with your shoulders.

2. Align your hips with your shoulders.

3. Tuck in the buttocks and bend your knees (slightly).

The pressure can be relieved when your body is resting if you sleep on a firm mattress. If you have a soft mattress; try placing a piece of plywood under it for a firmer surface.

Lifting Techniques: You should lift your back straight as you bring yourself up with your legs and hips. Hold the object close to your hips. You can also relieve some of the back pressure by using this technique.

Why Sciatica Happens

Sciatic nerve pain can have an effect on active or inactive people. The problem seems to be more common in men than women, and it usually plagues people over the age of 30.

Herniated Disc

A herniated or ruptured disk is one of the most common causes of sciatica. When a crack or tear develops on the disk, it bulges into the spinal canal (via a pinched sciatic nerve). It is estimated that one to two percent of every adult will have an experience with sciatic nerve pain.

Piriformis Syndrome

This syndrome develops when the small muscle that is deep within the buttocks (the piriformis muscle) spasms or becomes tight. This spasm produces irritation and pressure on the sciatic nerve.

Spinal Stenosis

The narrowing of open spaces in the spinal canal places

pressure on the nerves which travel through the spine to your arms and legs. The pain usually affects the neck and lower back. It is common with the aging population, usually individuals over 60 years old, and can also cause chronic sciatica pain.

Isthmic Spondylolisthesis

Your vertebra (the bone in your back) slips, so it is out of alignment with the vertebra above it because of a small stress fracture in a piece of the bone that connects the two joints on the back side of the spinal segment. The slippage causes a narrowing of the opening where the nerve lies.

Bone Spurs

An overgrowth bone (bone spur) can pinch the spinal nerve in the lower spine. The presence of spurs is an indication of spine degeneration which can begin in early adulthood but might not present until you reach the 60s or 70s age group. These factors can accelerate the degenerative process:

- Nutrition

- Heredity

- Traumatic Forces (including Motor vehicle accidents and sports injuries)

- Lifestyle (poor ergonomics and poor posture)

Degenerative Disc Disease

This is also referred to as DDD or osteoarthritis of the spine, and is actually not a disease—but a part of the aging process because of a loss of fluid in the tiny cracks and discs in the outer layer of the disc. It occurs most commonly in the lumbar region and the neck. The degenerated disc will lead to irritation resulting in irritation of the nerve root—thus sciatica.

Sacroiliac Joint Dysfunction and Sciatica

If your sacroiliac joint becomes inflamed, a portion of the sciatic nerve can also be irritated because it runs directly in front of the sacroiliac joint. However, the two issues have the same symptoms, but the pain caused by the sacroiliac joint isn't because of a compressed nerve root as it exits the spine—as with 'true sciatica.'

Doctor Appointment Preparation

Before you begin any plan, your physician will need to obtain a complete medical history as well as a review of your symptoms. You can get a jump start be preparation as shown below:

- Make a complete list of your symptoms and the dates when they began.

- Make another list of your key medical information including other existing conditions, as well as a list of all of your medications whether they are prescribed or over-the-counter. Be sure to include all supplements or vitamins you are taking.

- Include any recent injuries or accidents that could have damaged your back.

- Take a friend or family member with you to the doctor. It will be easier for two people to recall everything that will be discussed.

- Make a detailed list of any questions you need to ask your doctor at the appointment.

Ask questions such as these for the radiating lower back pain

- Do I need a diagnostic test?

- Are there other possible causes?

- What is the most likely cause of the pain in my back?

- What treatment do you recommend for me?

- What side effects will any prescribed medication cause?

- How long do I need to continue taking the medication?

- Is the medicine addictive?

- Am I considered a good candidate for surgery?

- Will there be any restrictions on me after surgery?

- What can I do to prevent recurrence of the problems?

Your Doctor's Response

- Do you have weakness or numbness in your legs?

- Are there specific activities or positions that cause your pain to become better or worse?

- Do you perform heavy/physical work?

- How good is your exercise plan? Do you have one? If yes, with what type of activities?

- What other treatments, if any, have your tried? Has anything helped with the sciatica pain?

During the physical exam, your physician will probably check your reflexes and muscle strength. You might be asked to walk on your toes or heels, lift your legs one at a time, or rise from a squatting position. He/ she may the refer you to other forms of tests to diagnose the problem.

Tests will be given to pinpoint the elevation when your pain begins to discover which nerves are affected and if you have any disc issues.

- Sciatica Diagnosis Procedures

Some of the tests might include:

- Electromyography

This testing (EMG/NCV) uses nerve conduction velocity to determine the electrical impulses which travel through your sciatic nerve. The test will usually clarify which nerve is being compressed—whether it is the buttock, back, or leg. The test can confirm whether the nerve compression is caused by spinal stenosis or a herniated disc.

X-Ray

The use of regular X-rays helps provide imaging to detect spinal fractures or changes in the spine such as a bone spur (bone overgrowth). One downside is that the X-ray doesn't provide a visual of the spine and soft tissues such as nerves, muscles, or the disc. It won't usually identify the cause of the symptoms.

Computed Tomography (CT)

If you have a CT scan performed, you may have a contrast

dye injected into the spinal canal before the X-rays are taken. The procedure is called a CT myelogram. Dye is injected between the vertebrae to diagnose whether a disc or vertebra is creating the painful symptoms. The dye will circulate around the spinal nerves and cord which will appear white on the scan.

Magnetic Resonance Imaging (MRI) Scans

The MRI will utilize a powerful magnet and computer system to provide three dimensions of all structures of the bone, muscles, spinal cord and nerves, the intervertebral disc, and other soft tissues.

For the MRI test, you will lie on a moving table into the MRI machine. The machine is loud, and your physician might consider giving you Valium (Diazepam) tablet to relieve some of the anxiety.

A successful treatment plan consists of three main components including personal training, massage, and acupuncture. Each of these elements will be fully explained.

3 - Sciatica Back Pain Relief

Sciatica treatment is meant to increase mobility and decrease pain. Many times the treatments for sciatica can include physical therapy, the use of medication for inflammation and pain, as well as limited rest using the floor or a firm mattress. Before you proceed with any type of new regimen, an accurate diagnosis should be made by your physician. You don't want to make the situation worse than it already is at this point. Proper diagnosis is also essential for these reasons:

- The exercise should be recommended by a physician for each specific case. The underlying cause of the pain must be discovered through various tests.

- Even though it is rare; other medical conditions can cause the sciatic pain including a fracture, tumor or other infections that might require prompt medical attention.

Medication

Anti-inflammatory drugs and pain medicines can help reduce stiffness and remedy the pain which can leave you ready for some exercise and allow you to become more mobile. As with many medications; you need to understand there might be some adverse side effects. You have several choices for your pain solutions:

Daily Vitamin Supplements for Sciatica

- B complex can speed healing.

- Bromelain (800 milligrams) naturally heals with anti-inflammatory medication to alleviate back pain.

- Calcium (2,000 milligrams) relieves nerve pressure and spasms.

- Magnesium (1,000 milligrams) helps relieve muscle spasms and nerve pressure.

- MSM (2,000 milligrams) is useful for general pain relief.

Non-Steroidal Anti-inflammatory Drugs (NSAIDs)

1. Aspirin (Not to be given to children 18 years old or younger because it will place him/her at increased

risk for Reye's Syndrome.

2. Naproxen (Aleve or Naprosyn)

3. Ibuprofen (Advil, Motrin IB, Rufen, and Nuprin)

4. Acetaminophen (Tylenol)

Prescription NSAIDS

1. Gabapentin (Neurontin) is a non-narcotic/anti-seizure drug which has successful treated sciatica.

2. Ibuprofen (Motrin)

3. Amitriptyline (Elavil)

4. Cyclobenzaprine (Flexeril)

5. Naproxen (Naprosyn and Anaprox)

6. Flurbiprofen (Ansaid)

7. Tizanidine (Zanaflex)

8. Meloxicam (Mobic)

9. Diclofenac (Voltaren)

Note: When taking NSAIDs it is advisable to take the medication with food to help reduce stomach discomfort. However, if you eat—it could slow down the pain-relief effect.

Antidepressants and Anti-Seizure Medications

- Amitriptyline

- Nortriptyline

Narcotics (Opiates/Opioids)

- Codeine

- Morphine

- Oxycodone

- Oxymorphone

- Hydrocodone

- Vicodin

Muscle Relaxants

- Diazepam

- Cyclobenzaprine

- Carisoprodol

- Methocarbamol

Note: Prescriptions might not be administered at the initial treatment time. It will depend on the level of pain. These are just some of the possible drugs that could be given if the physician believes any of them will benefit you.

Biofeedback Therapy

Although research has not been able to pinpoint why or how the biofeedback process works—it just does—it promotes relaxation. Electrodes are attached to your skin or finger sensors are used during a session. The sensors send signals to a monitor which will provide an image, flash, sound, or light to represent your skin temperature, blood pressure, breathing rate, sweating, or muscle activity.

The functions will change when you are under stress. The procedure is typically performed in a doctor's office, but some computer programs can be connected to our home computer. A biofeedback therapist will help you practice the relaxation exercises to focus on our sciatica pain. Some of the exercises include:

Guided Imagery

The procedure will cause you to focus your mind on a particular image (for example, the color and texture of a peach) to become more relaxed.

Mindfulness Meditation

The process will allow you to release negative emotions and place focus on your thought pattern.

Progressive Muscle Relaxation

The alternate tightening and relaxing of different muscle groups can help with the pain.

Deep Breathing

Breathing evenly allows you to calm your mind.

You can eventually learn how to control these functions on your own without the biofeedback equipment.

Physical Therapy and Yoga

You are probably asking, 'What's the Difference?' There is a unique difference between both methods. Please refer to some of the exercises provided to help you with the discomfort and pain.

Physical Therapy

Exercise movements given during physical therapy set the pace so you can reach the goal of not having so much pressure on the nerve. Special exercises may be given to you by the therapist to strengthen the muscles in your legs, abdomen, and back.

Physical therapists (PTs) are just that—someone who performs therapy. Passive techniques are performed to help with muscle relaxation. PTs are beneficial for rehab from surgery or with injuries. The PTs could benefit your pain management program.

Manual physical therapy can benefit those who have a sacroiliac joint dysfunction which also affects those with sciatica pain. The following types of movement are used for physical therapy techniques:

Soft Tissue Work

The process includes massage which will apply pressure to muscles (soft tissue). Circulation can be improved as the pressure relaxes the muscles and eases the pain.

Mobilization/Manipulation:

This method uses varying speeds (slow to fast) of measured movements, force (gentle to forceful), and distances (also called 'amplitude') where the joints are pulled, pushed or twisted to place the joints and bones into the correct positions. Flexibility and alignment are improved when the tight muscles are loosened around a joint.

Yoga

Yoga is also beneficial, but the skill is used on a whole person model. A yoga therapist is trained to work with muscular imbalances. Their training is in anatomy and the understanding of how different movement patterns can motivate healing processes.

Yoga therapists also teach you how to 'breathe through' the pain. The healing potential can be optimized with a yoga professional and working through comforting mental states through meditation.

Spinal Injections

The swelling and inflammation of the nerve roots can be remedied with the use of a cortisone-like anti-inflammatory medicine. Epidural steroid injections (ESIs and/or nerve blocks can help eliminate some of the pain when other conservative methods no longer remedy the severe pain.

Steroids such as prednisone or cortisone are used for the injection medication. If the pain doesn't recede after about a month or if other therapies haven't been successful, an x-ray guided injection might be a temporary fix.

The process has been used since 1952 and is still part of the non-surgical management plan or sciatica pain relief. The medicine is delivered directly/close to the source of the pain generation by 'flushing out' inflammatory chemicals and proteins from the local area.

In some cases, the injection alone is not sufficient but can be used combined with a comprehensive rehabilitation program. The effects tend to be temporary, but the relief can last from one week to one year. The injection can provide sufficient comfort so you can perform some of the stretching and exercises which can help with the process.

Unfortunately, because of side effects including loss of bone density, epidural shots are limited to three in a year. Check with your doctor about any updated limits on the process.

Surgery

In some cases, if conservative treatments aren't the solution to the severe pain and progressing symptoms—surgery might be the only option. Many physicians will consider surgery after four to six weeks of unremitting symptoms.

Surgery may also be indicated if the patient's ability to participate in daily activities is very limited. Surgery only becomes urgent if the patient has experienced progressive loss weakness in the legs or if bladder or bowel control has become an issue. Some of those options include:

Microdiscectomy

This procedure is used in cases where there has been a lumbar disc herniation. A small open surgery using magnification will remove the herniated disc fragments. This is a common surgical approach where the rest of the disc is left intact and is minimally invasive surgery.

Some doctors report patients who had this procedure experienced huge decreases in disability issues (approximately 90%), and pain for up to four years.

Discectomy

The simple meaning of discectomy means "cutting out the disc." The procedure is an "open" technique where a large skin incision is used along with a muscle retraction so the entire area can be viewed by the surgeon. The surgeon accesses the disc from the posterior (back) of the spine—

through the bone and muscles. Anywhere along the spine from cervical (the neck) to lumbar (low back) areas can be cut. Each case is different, but one or more of the disc can be removed.

The spine can be stabilized for those who have spinal instability, perform heavy labor or those who are athletes be receiving a fusion at the time of the discectomy. A fusion can use a combination of bone grafting or hardware (plates/screws) to connect the two vertebrae together.

As time passes, the healing process will allow the two vertebrae to refuse into one piece of bone. However, fusion is rarely necessary for a herniated lumbar disc. Posterior lumbar discectomy can be a helpful treatment plan for sciatica relief from a degenerative disc or a bulging/herniated disc.

Directly after surgery, a narcotic medication is usually prescribed but is limited to a two to four week period because the pain (narcotic) pills are very addictive. Pain is usually managed with other types of medication.

Laminectomy

For patients who suffer from lumbar spinal stenosis, this procedure might be recommended. The process includes removal of the lamina (the bone that covers the spinal cord) and the tissue/disc material which is the cause of pressure on the nerve.

The open decompression (lumbar laminectomy) differs from the microdiscectomy because there is more muscle stripping and the incision is longer. The midline of the back will be approached with a two to five-inch-long incision.

At multiple levels, on both sides (left and right), muscles (erector spinae) are dissected. After the spine is reached, the lamina is then removed, allowing the nerve root exposure. The facet joints (directly over the roots' nerve, can be trimmed (undercut) to give the nerve roots more space.

After the procedure, it is reported that 70 to 80% of patients have the ability to perform daily activities, and the level of discomfort and pain is reduced. However, because in the case of lumbar stenosis, created by arthritis ridden facet joints, the degenerative process may—after several years—

return.

4 - Sciatica Basic Exercises

It is important to remain physically active, even though it is probably the last thing you want to do if you are plagued by sciatica. Lying around can increase the chances of the pain remaining with you indefinitely.

For acute pain from sciatica, you are usually recommended to proceed with only light stretching a minimal exercise. If you have a bulging disc present in the lumbosacral area or a slipped/herniated disc, it is very important to strengthen the muscles to remove the lower back pressure and strain. With stronger muscles, the better you can expect to do what they do best—support your entire body.

Use the Correct Process

It is essential to exercise correctly. It is advisable to use the proper form or technique because without the right process; you could create increased or continued pain. Learn the exercises under the guidance of a trained healthcare practitioner such as a physiatrist, therapist, or chiropractor.

Simple Exercise

The key element is to keep moving. Try taking a 15- to 20-

minute walk because walking has a relatively low-impact on the lower back but has aerobic qualities. Try to escalate with a brisk pace up to three miles daily. Water aerobics might be a fun way to ease the pain, and swimming is an excellent way to apply all of your muscles.

The Pigeon Pose

The pigeon exercise is a common yoga pose which words to open the hips using multiple versions of stretching movements.

The reclining position is the most appropriate for a treatment beginner.

1. While lying on your back, bring up your right leg at a right angle while you lock your fingers behind your thigh.

2. Place your ankle against your knee while you grasp your left leg.

3. Hold the position briefly before switching legs. You are helping stretch the piriformis muscles which can press against the sciatic nerve.

4. Repeat the procedure after you switch sides and work the same process with the other leg.

The sitting position is a bit more difficult to accomplish

1. Sit on the floor with your legs in front of you. Begin by bending your right leg, and placing your right ankle on the top of your left knee.

2. Lean your upper body thigh. Hold the position for 15 to 30 seconds. Switch sides. You will discover this stretches the lower back and the glutes.

The forward pose uses a similar technique

1. Get on all fours in the floor (doggie-style).

2. Pick the right leg up and move it forward until the lowered leg is on the floor—horizontal to your body. With your knee to the right, place the right foot in front of your left knee.

3. With your toes pointed back and the top of your foot

on the ground, stretch your left leg behind you—all the way behind you.

4. Gradually, shift your body weight from your arms and legs until your legs are supporting your body. Sit straight up with your hands to either side of the legs.

5. Breathe deeply.

6. Exhale, while you lean over the upper body (forward) over your lower leg. Try to support the body weight with your arms as much as you can.

Hamstring Stretch While Standing

This standing/stretch will help relieve some of the tightness caused by sciatica:

1. While standing, (of course), use an elevated surface and put your right foot below—or at your hip level. Use a step on a stairway, an ottoman, or a chair as an elevation point. Try to keep a slight bend at the knee if it tends to become hyperextended.

2. Lean over as you bend your body slightly forward to-

ward your foot. Don't push too far to cause pain; you only want to feel the deep stretch.

3. Release your hip (of the raised leg) downward. You can use an exercise band or yoga strap under the left foot and over the right thigh for extra support.

4. Hold for a minimum of 30 seconds.

5. Repeat the exercise on the other side.

Knee to Opposite Shoulder Exercise

This exercise should help relieve the muscle, not cause pain.

1. Lay down on your back.

2. Extend your legs outward with your feet flexed upward.

3. Clasp the hands around the knee and gently pull the right leg across the body toward the left shoulder.

4. Hold the position for 30 seconds.

5. Push your knee to return to the starting position.

6. Repeat three times and switch legs.

Spinal Sitting Stretch

As the vertebrae in the spine compresses, sciatica pain is triggered. Try this exercise:

1. Sit on the floor with your feet flexed upward and your legs extended straight in front of you.

2. Place your right foot flat and bend your knee to the floor on the outside of your left knee.

3. Put your left elbow on the outside of your right knee as you turn gently to the right with your body.

4. Hold the position for about 30 seconds.

5. Repeat the exercise three times.

6. Lastly; Use the learned stretch with your left leg bent while you are turned onto your left side. Do you feel the stretch?

Low Lunge

1. Begin the stance in a runner's lunge position. Your right leg will be forward with the knee over your ankle and the left knee placed on the floor (foot flat on the floor). What a stretch!

2. Slowly, rest your hands on your right thigh as you slowly lift your torso.

3. Lean your hips slightly forward while you keep the right knee behind your toes.

4. Hold the position.

5. For a deeper stretch, raise your arms over your head (biceps by the ears). Hold for a minimum of 30 seconds.

6. Repeat the stretches on the opposite side.

"Cow's Face" Reclining Pose

This yoga pose might bring back childhood memories when it was much simpler to imitate a ball!

1. While on the floor—face-up—left leg over the right.

2. Flex both feet while raising both legs off of the floor

3. Hug your legs toward your belly as you reach up for the outer side of your ankle.

4. Keep your feet flexed and spread your toes as you gently hold your legs for a few breaths.

5. Switch to the opposite side and repeat the procedure.

Frog Pose

You might need to be in good physical shape for this one if you can obtain the pose; it does help:

1. Get on all fours (like a pup) with the knees on a blanket/mat (for comfort), and palms on the floor.

2. You want to feel the stretch of your inner thighs as you slowly widen your knees. You need to keep your foot and calf in contact with the floor.

3. Keep the ankles in line with your knees.

4. Lower down to your forearms.

5. Hold the position for 30 seconds.

Hip Rotation with a Foam Roll

This one is a crowd pleaser:

1. Place your feet flat on the floor—bent knees—and sit on the foam roller.

2. Place your right hand on the floor and lean your torso back.

3. Shift weight into the right hip and cross the right ankle over the left thigh.

4. Use the supporting hand and foot to roll from the bottom of your glutes to your pelvic bone.

5. Roll continuous for approximately 30 to 60 seconds.

Swiss Ball Leg Exercises

Balance the Ball Bridge:

1. Lay down on the ground with a balance ball under the

calves.

2. Keep the shoulders and neck on the ground as you raise the pelvis, so your upper legs and back are in a completely (or close) in a straight line.

3. Slowly, drop your pelvis to the ground.

4. Repeat the exercise 10 to 15 times.

Note: You can use a chair if you don't have a balance ball.

Balance Ball: The Diagonal Arm/Leg Raise

1. Lay down on your stomach while on the balance ball —arms and legs on the ground—a shoulder width apart.

2. Raise your left leg and right arm horizontally with the floor.

3. Hold for about 5 seconds—release—repeat on the other side.

Note: You can perform this exercise on our hands and knees

if you don't have access to a balance ball.

5 - Sciatica Exercises for Specific Issues

Herniated Disc

For many patients, press-ups or extension exercises can help with moving the pain from the leg to the lower back (which is a relief to some).

Herniated Disc Exercise

Lie on the floor (prone position) as if you are watching television with your elbows propping the upper body while our hips remain on the ground. This might be difficult, so proceed carefully and slowly. Not all patients are successful with this position at the beginning of exercise plans.

- Hold the position for approximately five seconds and work up to about 30 seconds for each repetition.

- Attempt to accomplish ten repetitions.

- After this position is mastered, try the advanced version:

- From the prone position, let your pelvis remain in

contact with the floor as you press up on your hands.

- Keep the buttocks and lower back relaxed to produce a gentle stretch

- Hold the position for one second.

- Repeat ten times.

Spinal Stenosis

Flexion exercises (forward bending techniques) are used by the spine specialist for sciatica from spinal stenosis. The size of the passageway is increased with the 'bending forward' movements which allow the impingement or irritation to resolve. For example, you might notice people using a cane, walker, or shopping cart walking; bent forward versus walking or standing up straight.

Specific exercises are necessary to strengthen and stretch which will focus on:

1. Stretching back muscles which hold the spine in proper extension (backward bending)

2. Strengthening of the muscles that bring the spine

into a forward bending position (flexion)

Spinal Stenosis Sciatica Stretching Exercises

Try to use the exercises below for the muscles in the lower back which keep and hold the spine in a bending backward position:

Back Flexion: Flexing

1. Lie down on your back and pull your knees gently to your chest until you begin to feel a comfortable stretch.

2. Hold for 30 seconds.

3. Slowly, return to the starting position.

4. Attempt to complete four to six repetitions of the flex.

Stretching

1. Sit on the floor on your hands and knees.

2. Sit back on your heels with your arms outstretched

and chest down.

3. Hold for 30 seconds.

4. Return slowly to the starting position.

5. Make an attempt to complete four to six repetitions of the stretch.

Tip: Don't bounce on the heels.

Degenerative Disc Disease

Several types of sciatica exercises are recommended for the degeneration of the disc will result in a dynamic lumbar stabilization program. Sometimes the McKenzie Method is used for the process.

The process involves locating the most comfortable position for the pelvis and lumbar spine—and training the body to maintain the position during all activities. If the exercise is done correctly, improvement will be shown through the sense of movement of the lumbar spine. It can also reduce the excess motion at each of the spinal segments which result in relieving pain and protecting the area from possible further damage.

Degenerative Disc Disease Exercises (On the Back)

Hook-Lying March:

1. Lay down with your back on the floor.

2. With bent knees and arms at your sides—tighten the stomach muscles.

3. Alternately—slowly raise your legs 3 to 4 inches off of the floor.

4. March for 30 seconds.

5. Repeat two to three times.

6. Take 30-second intervals between the repetitions.

Hook-Lying March Combination

Use the same method as used with the regular march (above), but add raising and lowering the opposite arm over your head.

Bridging

1. Lie on your back with bent knees.

2. Slowly, raise your buttocks from the floor.

3. Hold the bridge for 8 to 10 seconds.

4. Slowly, lower to the starting position.

As your skill and strength build; attempt to complete two sets of ten bridges.

Each of the exercises—the Hook-Lying March—the Hook-Lying March Combination—and the Bridging should be conducted with a rigid trunk. The pelvic tilt (with the buttocks flat on the floor and the tightening of your lower stomach muscles) can be used to locate the most comfortable position for your lower back.

Degenerative Disc Disease Exercises: On the Stomach

You will be using the same pelvic position (tightening stomach muscles to flatten the lower part of your back) to perform the sustaining exercises from lying flat on your stomach, as were used while on your back.

Exercise 1

1. With your knee slightly bent, raise one leg behind your knees, with no arch in the neck or back.

2. Hold the position for 4 to 6 seconds.

3. Slowly, lower your body to the starting position.

Attempt to do two sets/ten leg raises as you become stronger with the exercise.

Exercise 2

1. Lay with your face down, your arms stretched above your head, and elbows straight above your head.

2. Raise one of your arms and the opposite leg 2 to 3 inches from the ground.

3. Hold the position for 4 to 7 seconds.

4. Slowly lower your body to the starting position.

As you improve, try to complete two sets of the opposite side-raises.

Degenerative Disc Disease Exercises: Four-Point Position

You can also do similar exercises using the four-point position (kneeling on your hands and knees), as you raise your legs and arms, only as high as you can to be in complete control. You will want to avoid twisting or sagging and keep the trunk stabilized.

Exercise 1

1. With your knees slightly bent, raise one leg behind you with no arch in the neck or back.

2. Hold for 4 to 6 seconds.

3. Slowly lower yourself back to the starting position.

Increase to two sets of ten raises as your strength builds over time.

Exercise 2: Advanced Version of Exercise 1

1. With your knees slightly bent, raise one leg with no arch in the neck or back.

2. Raise the opposite arm.

3. Hold for 4 to 6 seconds.

4. Slowly, assume the start position.

As you become improved, it will be much easier to do at least two complete sets of ten leg raises.

Isthmic Spondylolisthesis

In most cases, isthmic spondylolisthesis affects the L5 nerve root. Most spine specialists will use hybrids of these two exercises:

- Stabilization programs used for treating degenerative disc disease

- Flexion based exercises used for treating spinal stenosis

These exercises require a 'hands-on' approach because if done incorrectly, you will not receive the full benefit of the exercise. Each of the exercises is much more difficult than they seem.

Pelvic Tilt

This exercise is useful to hold the spine in a flexed position.

1. Lie on your back with your knees bent and tighten the stomach muscles to flatten the body.

2. Pull the navel in and up.

3. Hold the pose for 10 to 20 seconds.

4. Relax the muscles.

Attempt to do a set of ten tilts for strengthening the lower stomach muscles.

Curl-Ups

You can help maintain a proper lower spine position while

strengthening the abdomen muscles with the curl-ups.

1. Lie down on your back with bent knees.

2. Fold your arms across your chest.

3. Tilt the pelvis to flatten your back by pulling the belly button (navel) in and up.

4. Lift your head and shoulders from the floor (Curl-Up). Tip: Don't make an attempt to lift too high.

5. Bring your head and chest toward the ceiling. Note for patients with cervical spine problems: Place your hands behind your head for extra support.

6. Hold for 2 to 4 seconds.

7. Slowly lower yourself to the start position.

As you strength sharpens, attempt to approach a minimum of two sets/ten curls.

Hook-Lying March

For an excellent stabilization exercise, the hook-lying march will help.

Note: See the exercise explained previously under the Degenerative Disc Disease section.

Piriformis Syndrome

The syndrome doesn't involve the disc extending beyond is usual location in the vertebral column—which technically isn't sciatica. However, the syndrome is the piriformis muscle itself that will irritate the sciatic nerve and cause the ensuing pain.

The piriformis muscle (previously described) is the muscle, very close to the sciatic nerve, which runs deep in the muscle of the hip. When the muscle becomes tightened and inflamed, it can cause sciatic nerve pain.

It's almost always essential—to relieve sciatic nerve pain—to stretch the piriformis muscle. Some of the same stretches are used for the hip extensor muscles and the hamstring muscles.

Piriformis Muscle Exercises: Stretches: Supine Piriformis Stretches

Exercise 1

1. Lie on your back with your legs flat on the floor.

2. Pull the affected leg up toward your chest while holding your knee (hand on the same side of your body); grasp the ankle with the other hand.

3. Attempt to lead with the ankle as you pull your knee toward the opposite ankle; you'll feel the stretch.

4. Hold the stretch for about 30 seconds.

5. Slowly return to the starting pose.

Set the goals to reach three sets of these stretches.

Exercise 2

1. Lie down on the floor—legs flat.

2. Slowly, raise the affected leg and place that foot on the ground outside of the opposite knee.

3. Gently, pull the knee of your bent leg directly across the midline of your body. (Use a towel or the opposite hand if needed.)

4. Try to hold the stretch for a minimum of 30 seconds.

5. Slowly, return to the starting pose.

Aim for a unit of three stretches.

Exercise 3

1. While on the floor; have your affected leg crossed over your other leg at our knees with both legs bent.

2. Gently pull your lower knee upwards toward our shoulder (on the same side of your body until you feel the stretch.)

3. Hold the stretch for approximately 30 seconds.

4. Lastly, return to the starting position.

Go for a complete set of three stretches.

Buttocks Stretch for the Piriformis Muscle

1. Assume the 'doggie-style' (on all fours) position.

2. Begin by placing the affected foot across and under the trunk of your body so the affected knee is outside of the trunk of your body.

3. Gently, extend the unaffected leg straight behind the trunk while you keep the pelvis straight.

4. At the same time, keep the affected leg in place; scoot your hips backward toward the ground while leaning forward on your forearms. Feel the stretch! Tip: Don't force your body to the floor.

5. Attempt to hold the stretch for about 30 seconds.

6. Slowly return to your starting pose.

Attempt to complete a set of three of these stretches.

Sacroiliac Joint Dysfunction and Sciatica: Single Knee to Chest Stretch

- While on your back—one at a time—pull one knee up to your chest while gently pumping the knee (upwards) 3 to 4 times at the top range of motion.

- Continue for ten repetitions for each leg.

Press-Up

- Get in the prone position (place your hands flat with your pelvis on the floor). Press up with your hands and hold the position for five seconds.

- Try to complete 10 repetitions.

Gradually increase to 30 seconds for each repetition.

Non-Weight Bearing—Lumbar Rotation

- Get onto your back and bend both knees.

- Keep your feet flat on the floor and rock your knees from side-to-side. Don't allow the knees to move very far apart and the thighs should rub together. The lower spine should remain basically still.

- Continue to rock the knees for about 30 seconds.

6 - Assisted Physical Remedies

It is best to take the natural approach when at all possible. Sciatica has endured a long and very painful history. Dating back to the 5th Century BC—sufferers and doctors alike—have attempted a host or remedies which varied from leeches to hot coals but in the 20th century, Roman times the use of injections and creams became a better option. You might also benefit from physical therapy or chiropractor adjustment to improve the nerve pain.

Chiropractic Treatments

A chiropractor can help your body heal on its own based on the scientific principal that restricted spinal movement can lead to reduced function, pain, and reduced performance. The type of method used may depend greatly upon the cause of the sciatica pain. Several treatments can be used including—but not limited to—ultrasound, ice/cold therapy, TENS, and spinal adjustments.

- Ultrasound

The use of ultrasound provides a relaxing heat created by sound waves to penetrate deep into your tissues. Circulation is improved, resulting in reduced swelling, cramping, muscle spasms, pain, and stiffness.

- Hot and Cold Therapy helps reduce inflammation and control pain.

- Transcutaneous Electrical Nerve Stimulation (TENS)

The TENS unit is a battery-powered, small box-like, portable muscle stimulating machine. The use of variable intensities of electrical current charges control and help reduce muscle spasms. The smaller version of the TENS unit is used at home, but a larger version is provided by physical therapists, chiropractors, and other similar rehabilitation professionals.

- Spinal Adjustments

Spinal adjustments also called spinal manipulations can sometimes be a good defense for relieving the sciatic nerve pressure. The procedure promotes the body's regular healing mechanisms.

According to a 2010 study in the Journal of Manipulative and Psychological Therapeutics, approximately 60% of the patients who received spinal manipulation experienced the same levels of pain relief as those who opted to have surgery.

With three to four visits each week, the research study revealed that with continued weekly visits, the treatment could be tapered off because of the satisfactory improvement.

Acupuncture and Cupping

Acupuncture can also use cupping or sliding whereas glass cups are placed on the body to create suction in the affected area. The blood flow is increased with the procedure so the muscles can relax and the pressure can be removed away from the sciatic nerve via the suction component.

The Chinese medicine practice—needling—has achieved many ways of opening your body's natural flow of energy. The tiny needles are virtually pain-free and able to target the disturbed pathways in your body. The FDA has approved its use for chronic pains including sciatica. Sometimes, electro-acupuncture is performed which sends a vibration down the length of the needle to reach the nerves pathway.

You can get some relief after the first session, but it could take about twelve sessions before you notice any major improvement. According to a Chinese study of 30 people with sciatica, 17 of the patients received complete relief and ten of them observed improvement with the use of acupuncture using heated needles (warming acupuncture).

Acupressure for Sciatic Pain Relief

Acupressure is similar to acupuncture in that is also used as an alternative medicine technique—with the means of pressure being the difference between the two methods.

Acupuncture uses needles, whereas acupressure uses physical pressure points over specific body points. Elbows, hands, or other devices can be used for the pressure tool. These are the two points of pressure to apply acupressure to for sciatica:

Point 1

Locate the GB-30 also called the acupoint Jumping Circle which is located midway between the right hipbone and the tip of the tailbone (coccyx) and is aligned with the center of the buttocks.

- Heavy pressure is applied using the index finger or right thumb until you feel the soreness.

- Hold for approximately 30 seconds.

- Release and repeat a few times as you alternate from the left and right sides.

Point 2

The pressure point behind the knee called the GB-34 or Yang Spring acupoint is on the outer part of the right/lower leg. It is near the end of the knee crease just below the bony structure about a four-finger width below the kneecap.

- Apply a constant/steady pressure with the right thumb until some soreness is felt.

- Hold for about 3 minutes.

- Repeat on the left leg.

These two pressure points are an excellent method for strengthening the tendons and relaxing while you treat sciatica at the same time.

Inversion Table

For individuals who want to avoid surgery, the use of an inversion table would benefit the sciatica pain. The table is a form of therapy involving the patient being upside down or at an inverted angle; while at the same time—hanging by the ankles, legs, or feet.

The inversion process is a form of spinal decompression or spinal traction. The traction elongates the spine by increasing the space between each vertebra which in turn relieves the pressure on the discs, nerve roots, and ligaments.

According to the Healthy Back Institute, most individuals will invert between 5 to 15 minutes—or—1 to 2 times daily. You can do it anytime, but listen to your body; it will know when you have had enough!

Massage Therapy

Your sciatic nerve roots can benefit from massage by loosening the tight lower back muscles surrounding the nerve and helps prevent irritation and pinching. It encourages the release of pain-fighting endorphins. An increased blood flow speeds healing to the area with fresh and oxygenated blood to a space where the flow had been compromised.

If you are in the 3rd trimester of pregnancy, a cyclist, or a runner—massage can help and is strongly recommended by therapists.

Rolfing

Rolfing is the process is called "the recipe" which was invented by Ida P. Rolf with the theory of how the human body's "energy field" can benefit you when it is aligned with the Earth's gravitational field. The recipe uses superficial to deep manual therapy which can sometimes become painful.

Rolfing benefits the body through soft tissue manipulation. It is unlike massage—which mainly focuses on relief and relaxation—Rolfing is working towards improving functioning and alignment.

Rolfing is also different from deep-tissue massage, in that the practitioners are trained to create balance and ease, rather than focusing on areas presenting with tension.

Lastly, Rolfing can speed up injury recovery by reducing stiffness, pain, and muscle tension. Therefore, you will begin to notice improved movement and circulation around the joints.

7 - Home Treatment and Natural Remedies

The cornerstone of treatment for sciatica is activity modification as well as pain medication. After you are properly diagnosed, your doctor will probably prescribe some form of medication to relieve your symptoms. However, you can also use some home remedies along with the medication to boost the healing process.

Rest

Sciatica pain can make life difficult, to say the least! Ample rest lying on a flat surface with a soft pillow underneath the knees should provide some comfort. After about two hours, alternate your position and sleep on your side. Be sure to keep your back straight (with the aid of the pillow between the legs).

Heating Pads and Heat Wraps

Several times daily you can use a heating pad on a low or medium setting for 15 to 20 minutes for a temporary bit of pain relief. It is a convenient way to achieve some relief whether you are at home or work. You can safely use the heating pad for two to three hours each day. Some heating pads are moist heat which seems to work better for pain relief. You can also purchase single-use heat wraps which will last for a specified amount of time.

If you don't have access to an electric heating pad; you can use a hand towel that has been run under hot water. Place it on the affected area and proceed with another hot towel when the first one gets cold using the same amount of time for treatment as you would for a heating pad. You could also place the towel briefly in the microwave, but be careful not to get it too hot.

Tip: For safety reasons don't attempt to go to sleep with the heating pad on your body. You could wake up with a severe burn.

Infrared Light

Purchase an infrared mat to help with some of the sciatica nerve pain. The process involves plugging the mat into an electrical source and lying flat on the mat. The nerve will become relaxed after the light has worked its magic.

Infrared heating pads use natural stones, such as Jade, to

deliver the deep penetrating heat that can penetrate to the levels needed for a uniform warming effect.

Warm Bath versus the Ice Pack

If the heating pad helps, you could also try a warm bath to loosen the tightened muscles and help increase circulation. You will also enjoy the bath!

Heat works well with many patients who suffer from sciatica pain. On the other hand, sometimes an ice pack works. The cold treatment will help reduce the swelling around the nerve and help numb the pain. If you don't have a cold pack, use a bag of frozen veggies.

If you have a partner or friend, have him/her use an ice cube in a triangular pattern around the affected/sore area. Try not to concentrate in one area, cover the entire space. If the area becomes to feel too cold, simply stop the process.

Choose the option that works best for you for 15- to 20-minute intervals. You can do this every two or three hours until you receive some relief.

Epsom Salts Bath

The magnesium mineral is crucial for you to have healthy nerve function. Epsom salt is a combination of sulfate and magnesium which is easily absorbed through the pores of your skin.

Use lukewarm water (body temperature) in a shallow bath.

1. Add 1 Cup Epsom Salts

2. Add 2 Tablespoons Eucalyptus Oil

3. Add a Few Drops of Chamomile Oil & Lavender Oil

4. Soak for 20 minutes to relax.

5. Take a lukewarm shower.

Bathe in the solution twice each day until the pain is relieved.

Or, if you choose to prepare a hot bath with just two cups of Epsom salt and enjoy the astonishing relief from your sciatica. Be sure to keep your legs and back submerged in the water for a minimum of 20 minutes. Use this bath for at least three times weekly for the best results.

Inflammation Reduction

Many of the risk factors for sciatic nerve pain can be caused by inflammation which can make healing time extensive for injuries and the inevitability of increased pain. You should also consider eating a nutrient-dense healing diet (See Chapter 7), avoid risky behaviors, and be sure to get plenty of sleep and exercise.

Ginger to the Rescue

Ginger is one of the most powerful natural nerve pain remedies invented thus far. Its anti-inflammatory elements are rich in potassium (a potassium deficiency is known to exacerbate sciatica pain). Try some of these healthy/natural methods:

Ginger Tea

- 1 Cup Boiled Water

- Add 2 or 3 slices Ginger (finely sliced)

- 1 Teaspoon of Ginger Powder

- 1 Teaspoon Natural Honey (to taste)

- Squeeze of Lemon Juice

Add the ingredients.

Let the tea steep until it is cool.

Drink 3 times daily on an empty stomach.

Ginger Slices

Purchase some dried ginger slices from the local health food store or online. Don't use the sugar coated ginger. Eat 8 to 10 slices each day; also on an empty stomach.

Chew Fresh Ginger

The chewing of ginger works but it is hot! Chew it until the juice is gone and spit it out. Don't swallow it! You can repeat the process during the day.

Beneficial Drinks

These are just a few of the ways to accomplish pain relief other than plain water:

Water and Juice

Drinking plenty of water (a minimum of eight-8 ounce glasses daily) not only helps reduce inflammation but it aids in lubricating the vertebrae in the spine. Call it the 8 x 8 rule if you cannot remember the number, it's catchy! If you prefer drinking tea or juice, try a tasty wild celery leaf—potato—beets—or carrot root for pain reduction.

When it comes to sciatica, the goal is to hydrate, to nourish your nerves, and reduce inflammation.

Astragalus Tea

This Chinese tea is exceptional for its antibacterial and anti-inflammatory elements. You can purchase the herb in tablets, capsules, or in liquid form. To make the tea:

1. Bring 1 Quart of water to a boil.

2. Add 4 Ounces of Fresh Astragalus Root or 3 to 5 Tablespoons of Dried Astragalus Root.

3. Boil the root for 3 to 4 minutes.

4. Strain the tea and remove any debris by using a coffee filter or cheesecloth.

5. Place the fresh tea in an air-tight container in the refrigerator.

Have a fresh mug now and later. You should attempt to drink two to four cups daily for immune support improvement.

Black Snakeroot

- Heat 1 Cup of Water

- Add; ½ Tablespoon of Dried Black Snakeroots

- Set aside for 15 minutes.

Drink 2 Tablespoons at least three times daily.

Burdock Root Tea

Burdock is a member of the aster family and can be consumed two or three times daily for sciatica relief.

Place some burdock root (you only need a pinch of the root) in water for 2 to 3 minutes. You can also purchase the burdock root in a tea bag or powder form.

Celery

As an antioxidant and anti-inflammatory source, celery consists of a compound known as coumarin (fragrant flavoring) which contains high concentrations of cinnamon.

1. Boil one glass/cup of water.

2. Add leaves and stems.

3. Boil until the water is green.

4. 3 cups to be drunk daily.

Chamomile Tea

The tea is a muscle relaxer and can be used to help relieve

the pain of sciatica. Steep the chamomile tea bags in a cup of water for 5 minutes. You can drink 3 cups each day.

Devil's Claw

This herbal medication is a potent anti-inflammatory which works similar to ibuprofen and other products in the same category. Generally, the dosage is set twice each day with dosages between 1,500 to 2,000 mg. Search for a brand that has the standardized extract of 50 mg of harpagoside, the active compound.

Tip: This should be avoided by patients with blood-thinning medications or peptic ulcers.

Elderberry Juice

All parts (leaves, fruit, and flowers) can be used for relaxing elements to reduce the pressure on your nerve endings. For the best results; drink a glass of elderberry just a minimum of two times daily

Fenugreek Seeds

- Overnight, soak 1 Teaspoon of Fenugreek Seeds.

- In the morning, strain the water.

- Drink on an empty stomach.

Potato Juice

This superb mixture assists the movement of your feet and legs by reducing the irritated sciatic nerve.

- Grate 1 raw potato & extract the juice.

- Mix the potato juice with some carrot juice.

Drink 2 times daily.

Turmeric

Try this healthy drink for a bit of relief:

- One Teaspoon Turmeric

- One Cup of Milk

- Add one teaspoon of turmeric to the milk.

- Boil the solution.

- If you desire, add a small cinnamon stick (you will at least enjoy the aroma).

Use honey as a sweetener and have this drink once or twice each day.

Valerian Root

Muscle spasms caused by sciatica pain can be remedied with valerian root. The root helps ease the tension and relax the muscles—another plus to aid with sleeping more comfortably. Consult with your doctor before you use either of these methods. Try valerian root one of these ways:

- Supplement: Take 150 mg of the valerian root supplement three times daily for several weeks.

- Valerian Tea: Use one cup of hot water and steep 1 Teaspoon of Dried Valerian Root for 10 minutes. You can drink this several times weekly for several weeks.

Other Hydration and Lubrication Methods: Massage

Have a friend or partner massage the affected area two or

three times a day using Saint-John's-Wort oil for a bit of relief. The anti-inflammatory, antioxidant, antibacterial, and astringent elements in the oil can help immensely. The yellow-flowered plant has been used for medicinal purposes since the ancient days of Greece.

Lemon Balm

Lemon balm is a strong aromatic herb which means you might need to use only half of the quantity for the herbal infusion. You can also enjoy frequent cups of tisane (aromatic tea which is steeped for only a few minutes similar to a tea bag). The balm will balance the nervous system and calms anxiety.

Licorice Root

As a great source of alleviating pain and swelling, you will love the aroma. Only a small amount (1 Tablespoon per quart) is necessary for an infusion.

Linden Flower/Leaf

Your nerves will love this plant! It is from the Malvaceae family which also has other beneficial flowers including the

Rose of Sharon, hibiscus, marshmallow, or okra.

Milky Oat Tops

Nerve restoration is given particularly with just the milky oat tops.

Tinctures/Elixir/Extract from Herbals

Willow Bark is used as is a classic for an anti-inflammatory pain reliever. However, it doesn't taste good, but it works.

Wild lettuce works for people in different ways. It is used as a sedative because of its sleep-inducing formula but is also a good pain reducer.

Black Birch is similar to Willow but has a better flavor. It is also useful to settle your stomach.

Herb-of-Grace or Common Rue is an ornamental plant but is also a herb. One patient stated he/she made a tincture of rue by using 3 drops—twice daily.

Mullein Root is used specifically for sciatica or for when you know your 'back is out' or something 'feels tweaked.' Use a 5 drop dose approximately three times each day.

Skullcap will produce a calming effect. This classic herb grows along riverbanks in its natural habitat. It can be found in tranquil shade and water.

Other Natural Anti-Inflammatory Muscle Relaxants

For the aching muscles, use some chamomile or celery seed.

You can try also try:

- Rosemary

- Grape seed extract

- Bromelain

- Angelica

Other Liniments and Oils

It has been proven that frequent applications of anti-inflammatory, nerve healing and muscle relaxing herbal infused oils will provide additional help. You can prepare the oils at home by steeping the herbs in a carrier oil for four to six weeks. If you are fortunate, you can purchase the oils from an apothecary or order them online.

Some of the best infusion oils include:

- Birch

- Brahmi (Gotu Kola)

- Goldenrod

- Yarrow

Some patients found using straight St. John's Wort infused oil to a small amount of Roman chamomile oil provided a great pain killing salve delivers directly to the muscle tissue and provides a warming sensation; whereas the St. John's Wort directs its elements to the primary nerves with a cooling effect.

Essential Oils are different than infused oils. A distillation process is most often used to obtain the pure volatile oil from plants. Each product is highly concentrated and must be carefully handled. Each plant has a special application process. You can dilute a few drops of your herbal infused oil.

Note: Essential oils are meant for external use only.

- Chamomile is an excellent anti-inflammatory produce and is excellent for soothing your spirit and body.

- Clary Sage is an excellent pain reliever and is used for muscle spasms and severe injuries.

- Lavender is comforting and healing to make you feel centered at home.

- Peppermint will increase your circulation with its cooling effects to reduce swelling without raising the heat. Use it on any part of your body that seems 'stuck.'

Other Remedies

Capsaicin Cream

Cayenne pepper is the active ingredient which works as a natural pain reliever. The levels of a neurotransmitter called substance 'P' transports the pain signals. The capsaicin ointment/cream helps block the signal. You can benefit from capsaicin which also comes in different strengths (0.025% up to 0.075%). Initially, you might notice a burning sensation.

Note: Don't apply to broken skin.

Garlic

You might be surprised, but garlic is also great for inflammation and can be used in many of your dishes. Four raw cloves every morning might be all you need to fight the daily pain. You can also choose to take a garlic supplement for relief.

Jamaican Dogwood

You may recognize the name of the Jamaican dogwood by other names—Piscidia erythrnia—fish-fuddle—or the Florida Fish-poison tree. The bark of the tree contains a powerful substance for nerve pain relief. It can be taken in the form of a supplemental capsule or applied as a tincture. However, the Jamaican dogwood should not be used by lactating or pregnant women.

Fenugreek Seeds Paste

1. Grind a few of the fenugreek seeds.

2. Boil the powder with enough milk to make a mushy paste.

3. Apply the paste/poultice to the area of pain.

4. Leave the mixture on for several hours before washing it off your skin.

Repeat the process each day until some relief is noted.

Horseradish Poultice

This is a simple home remedy which should provide you with some pain relief. Here is the method:

1. Grind ½ of Horseradish Root into a paste.

2. Apply the paste to a warm cloth.

3. Cover the area for up to one hour to relieve the nerve pain and neuropathies.

Burdock Root Mixture

Place some burdock root powder in water for 15 to 20 minutes.

Use a cotton cloth soaked in the burdock mixture and apply it to the area.

Mustard Oil Mixture

1. Heat 3 Tablespoons of Mustard Oil

2. Add; 3 Crushed Cloves of Garlic

3. Add; A few carom seeds to the mix.

4. Allow the oil to cool.

Massage onto the affected areas.

Nutmeg Powder Mixture

1. Roast a small amount of nutmeg powder in 1 Table-spoon of Ginger Oil.

2. Let the mixture cool.

3. Apply to the affected area.

Over-the-Counter Medications

If natural remedies don't seem to help eliminate your pain,

many doctors recommend Ibuprofen/Advil or Tylenol.

8 - Diet Planning and Inflammation

Inflammation can sometimes be reduced if you simply watch your diet. As with any diet, it is best to speak with your doctor to search for natural foods with a nutrition enriched diet plan to help you treat sciatica.

Many fruits including fresh pineapple and berries of all sorts contain anti-inflammatory aid to promote healing and also enhance the immune system.

These are just a few of the food products you can consume to help improve your sciatica pain through your diet choices:

Magnesium

Magnesium enriched foods help release muscle contractions. Magnesium supplements can be taken, but it is a powerful pill and should be taken in dosages of 600 to 800 mg daily. (Beware of possible side effects and notify your doctor.) You can also find magnesium in:

- Apples

• Apricots

• Brown rice

• Dairy products

• Seafood

• Lima beans

• Dulse (Seaweed that tastes like bacon)

Halibut contains many useful ingredients/nutrients including protein, omega-3 fatty acids, vitamins B3, B6, and B-12, selenium, tryptophan, and phosphorus. The B-12 is especially significant to treat your sciatic nerve pain.

Potassium

Controlled portions of potassium can help ward off sciatic nerve pain. Physicians recommend taking 4.7 grams of potassium daily for women and men. Be advised; it could take up to two weeks before you see considerable changes in the sciatica pain. These are some of the products which are helpful in the potassium category:

- Avocados: One ounce

- Baked Potato: One

- Bananas: One cup

- Cantaloupe: One Cup

- Chlorella (single-cell green algae)

- Cooked Beets: One cup

- Dried Apricots: 10 halves

- Honeydew Melons: One cup

- Plain Yogurt: One cup

- Raw Kiwi: One

- Raw Nectarines: One

- Raw Oranges: One

- Raw Pears: One

- Lima Beans: One cup

- Orange Juice: One cup

- Peanuts: One ounce

- Skim Milk: 8 ounces

- Spirulina (freshwater plant)

- Tomato Products

- Winter Squash: One Cup

B Vitamins can also help relieve pain through these products:

- Cheese

- Clams

- Lamb

- Liver

- Oysters

- Green Peas

- Navy beans

- Pinto beans

- Wheat Bran

- Spinach

- Sweet potatoes

- Soy Beans

- Bananas

- Nuts

- Whole grain fortified breads and cereals

- Unpolished rice and legumes

- Sunflower Seeds

- Peanut Butter

Vitamin A

- Dairy Products: Cheese, Milk, Yogurt

- Dark leafy green vegetables

- Carrots

- Orange colored fruits

- Apricots

- Mangoes

- Fortified margarine

- Mackerel and other oily fish

- Eggs

Vitamin C

- All fruits (More found in citrus)

- Regular and Sweet Potatoes

- Spinach

- Cabbage

- Broccoli

- Green veggies

- Yellow veggies

- Tomatoes

Vitamin K

- Alfalfa

- Broccoli

- Spinach

- Vegetable oils

Antioxidants

- Spices such as ginger, turmeric, and garlic are excellent sources of antioxidants.

- Green Tea: 2 – 3 cups per day with its fabulous antioxidant properties

- Turmeric

Beef: Grass-fed beef (Eaten in moderation)

Black Beans

- Kidney Beans

- Soybeans

Fiber-Enriched Foods

- Many fruits and vegetables will prevent constipation.

Omega 3 Fatty Acids

- Oily fish such as salmon, sardines, herrings and mackerel, and halibut-rich in omega 3 fatty acids.

- Include walnuts, canola oil, and flaxseeds

Bad Foods for Sciatica Sufferers

Added Sugars

Ingredients that will add calories and a sweet flavor—but few nutrients—are the added sugars to avoid if you suffer from sciatica. These sugars are also unhealthy because they are high-glycemic (high impact on blood sugar levels). Increased inflammation can be caused by the products—junk food—that is so enjoyable; versus the veggies and fruits which are beneficial.

Avoid these products

- Commercially prepared products such as brownies, pies, cakes, or cookies

- Sweetened cereals

- Regular soft drinks

- Pancake syrup

- Candy

- Frosting

- Frozen

- Desserts

(There went the rest of the goodies).

Refined Grains

Whole grains should be chosen over refined grains because

of the process used to create the refined products have been stripped of valuable nutrients, including the B-vitamins. To promote sufficient fiber intake and receive sufficient nutrients, whole grain is the best choice.

These are some of the products to avoid:

- Low-fiber cereals

- Baked goods prepared with white cake or baking flour

- White bread

- Instant rice

- Enriched pasta

(There went the morning donuts).

Saturated Fat

Inflammation is increased with the use of saturated fats. According to the American Heart Association, the diet plan should contribute less than 7% of your daily calorie limits to saturated fats.

Some of the sources include:

- Fried foods

- Egg yolks

- Red Meats

- Processed meats

- Poultry skin

- Dark-meat poultry

- High-fat dairy products

Trans-Fats

You may also have heard the chemically-produced fats are also called trans-fatty acids. Either way, you can increase the LDL (bad) cholesterol, and lower the HDL (good) cholesterol.

Sources included are:

- Shortening and commercial foods which list hydrogenated vegetable oil as an ingredient

- Stick Margarine

9 - Conclusion

Firstly, I would like to take this opportunity to thank you for downloading this book, Sciatica: Pain Relief Guide: Exercise —Back Pain Relief—Natural Remedies & Home Treatment.

For people who suffer from sciatic pain, with plenty of rest and time approximately 80 to 90% can improve without surgical procedures. Many can recuperate from a sciatic episode within six weeks.

I hope the data from Sciatica was a helpful aid so you could discover some of the reasons you suffer from the misery involved with sciatica pain whether you are walking, sitting, or standing. Pain can become chronic and lead to disabilities with some people. Sciatica also tends to have frequent recurrence rates, sometimes with no warning.

The next step is for you to decide which path you will take for symptom relief. Remember how important it is to avoid movements during recovery times including twisting your back and bending at the same time. It is the small things that can cause sciatica flare-ups. Hopefully, with this information, the choices have become much clearer.

You can do it! After all, look at this list of famous people with sciatica.

Do you know any of them?

- Debbie Allen: An American dancer and choreographer.

- James Cagney: An American stage and film actor.

- Duncan Ferguson: A Scottish ex-footballer who played for Everton and Newcastle United.

- Eileen Joyce: An Australian concert pianist.

My greatest joy is that you enjoyed Sciatica: Pain Relief Guide: Exercise—Back Pain Relief—Natural Remedies & Home Treatment.

Thanks again and good luck with your pain!

Thank You

As we reach the end of this book, I want to say thanks for reading this book.

I want to get this information out to as many people as possible. If you found this book helpful, I would greatly appreciate you leaving me a review on Amazon here. This helps others find the book as well.

I love hearing from readers so please get in touch via E-mail: cabpublishing1@gmail.com[1]

------

[1] mailto:cabpublishing1@gmail.com

Disclaimer

This document is geared towards providing exact and reliable information in regards to the topic and issue covered. The publication is sold with the idea that the publisher is not required to render accounting, officially permitted, or otherwise, qualified services. If advice is necessary, legal or professional, a practiced individual in the profession should be ordered.

This information is not presented by a medical practicioner and is for educational and informational purposes only. The content is not intended as a substitute for professional medical advice, diagnosis, or treatment. Always seek the advice of your physician or other qualified health care provider with any questions you may have regarding a medical condition. Never disregard professional medical advice or delay in seeking it because of something you have read.

The information provided herein is stated to be truthful and consistent, in that any liability, in terms of inattention or otherwise, by any usage or abuse of any policies, processes, or directions contained within is the solitary and utter responsibility of the recipient reader. Under no circumstances will any legal responsibility or blame be held against the

DISCLAIMER

publisher for any reparation, damages, or monetary loss due to the information herein, either directly or indirectly.

Last Updated: 08.Sep.2016